ACL Injuries in Female Athletes

ACL Injuries in Female Athletes

ROBIN WEST, MD
Chairman
Sports Medicine
Inova Health System
Fairfax, VA, United States

Associate Professor
Department of Orthopaedics
Georgetown Univeristy Medical Center
Washington, DC, United States

Head Team Physician
Washington Redskins
Ashburn, VA, United States

Lead Team Physician
Washington Nationals
Washington, DC, United States

BRANDON BRYANT, BS, MD
Orthopedic Sports Medicine Surgeon
Orthopedic Sports Medicine
Inova Orthopedics and Sports Medicine
Fairfax, VA, United States

ELSEVIER

ELSEVIER

3251 Riverport Lane
St. Louis, Missouri 63043

ACL Injuries in Female Athletes   ISBN: 978-0-323-54839-7

Publisher: Mica Haley
Acquisition Editor: Kayla Wolfe
Editorial Project Manager: Barbara Makinster
Project Manager: Kiruthika Govindaraju
Designer: Alan Studholme

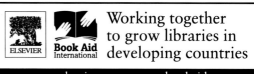

Working together to grow libraries in developing countries

www.elsevier.com • www.bookaid.org

List of Contributors

Marcio Albers, MD
Research Fellow
Orthopaedic Surgery
University of Pittsburgh, Pittsburgh
Pittsburgh, PA, United States

John P. Begly, MD
Orthopedic Sports Medicine Fellow
The Steadman Clinic
Vail, CO, United States

Kieran R. Bhattacharya, BCh
Medical Student
Orthopaedic Surgery
University of Virginia School of Medicine
Charlottesville, VA, United States

Seth Blee, MSPT, DPT, CFMT, CSCS
Regional Clinic Director
Physical Therapy
Inova Physical Therapy Center
Fairfax, VA, United States

Physical Therapist
Washington Nationals
Washington, DC, United States

Primary Faculty Member
Institute of Physical Art
Steamboat Springs, CO, United States

Brandon Bryant, BS, MD
Orthopedic Sports Medicine Surgeon
Orthopedic Sports Medicine
Inova Orthopedics and Sports Medicine
Fairfax, VA, United States

Monique C. Chambers, MD, MSL
Academic Health Sciences Fellow
Orthopedic Surgery
University of Pittsburgh
Pittsburgh, PA, United States

Edward S. Chang, MD
Assistant Professor
Orthopedic Surgery
Inova Health System
Fairfax, VA, United States

Assistant Professor
Orthopedic Surgery
Virginia Commonwealth University School of Medicine
Fairfax, VA, United States

James D. Doorley, MA
Doctoral Student
Psychology
George Mason University
Fairfax, VA, United States

Freddie H. Fu, MD, DSc (Hon), DPs (Hon)
Distinguished Service Professor
University of Pittsburgh
Pittsburgh, PA, United States

David Silver Professor and Chairman
Department of Orthopaedic Surgery
University of Pittsburgh School of Medicine
Pittsburgh, PA, United States

Head Team Physician
Athletics
University of Pittsburgh
Pittsburgh, PA, United States

Bryan L. Goldstein, BA
Hiram College
Hiram, OH, United States

Brendan T. Higgins, MD, MS
Orthopedic Sports Medicine Fellow
The Steadman Clinic
Vail, CO, United States

Christopher D. Joyce, MD
University of Colorado School of Medicine
Aurora, CO, United States

Meredith Mayo
Stanford University
Aurora, CO, United States

Patrick Wakefield Joyner, MD, MS
Doctor
Orthopaedic Sports Medicine
Naples Orthopaedics & Sports Medicine
Naples, FL, United States

Ajay Kanakamedala, MD
Research Fellow
Orthopaedic Surgery
University of Pittsburgh
Pittsburgh, PA, United States

Michelle E. Kew, MD
Resident
Orthopaedic Surgery
University of Virginia
Charlottesville, VA, United States

Mininder S. Kocher, MD, MPH
Professor of Orthopaedic Surgery
Orthopaedic Surgery
Harvard Medical School
Boston, MA, United States

Associate Director
Division of Sports Medicine, Department of
    Orthopaedic Surgery
Boston Children's Hospital
Boston, MA, United States

Marcin Kowalczuk, MD
Department of Orthopaedic Surgery
University of Pittsburgh
Pittsburgh, PA, United States

Pamela J. Lang, MD
Assistant Professor
Department of Orthopedics and Rehabilitation
University of Wisconsin School of Medicine and
    Public Health
Madison, WI, United States

Meredith Mayo, MD
Meredith Mayo
Stanford University
Aurora, CO, United States

Mark D. Miller, MD
Orthopaedics
University of Virginia
Charlottesville, VA, United States

Volker Musahl, MD
Assistant Professor
Orthopaedic Surgery
University of Pittsburgh
Pittsburgh, PA, United States

Colin P. Murphy, BA
Steadman Philippon Research Institute
Vail, CO, United States

Miguel A. Pelton, MD
Orthopaedic Surgery
Georgetown University Hospital
Washington DC, United States

Matthew T. Provencher, MD, CAPT, MC, USNR
Orthopaedic Clinic
The Steadman Clinic
Vail, CO, United States

Scott A. Rodeo, MD
Professor of Orthopaedic Surgery (Academic Track)
Weill Medical College of Cornell University
Ithaca, NY, United States

Co-Chief, Sports Medicine and Shoulder Service
Hospital for Special Surgery
Attending Orthopaedic Surgeon
Hospital for Special Surgery
Ithaca, NY, United States

Anthony Sanchez, BS
Steadman Philippon Research Institute
Vail, CO, United States

Lee Sasala, MD
Department of Orthopaedic Surgery
University of Pittsburgh
Pittsburgh, PA, United States

Andrew J. Sheean, MD
Physician
Orthopaedic Surgery
University of Pittsburgh
Pittsburgh, PA, United States

Andrea M. Spiker, MD
Assistant Professor
Orthopedic Surgery
University of Wisconsin–Madison
Madison, WI, United States

Genevra L. Stone, MD
Beth Israel Deaconess Medical Center
Boston, MA, United States

Eleonor Svantesson, MD, PhD
Department of Orthopaedic Surgery
Institute of Clinical Sciences
The Sahlgrenska Academy
University of Gothenburg
Gothenburg, Sweden

Armando F. Vidal, MD
Associate Professor
Department of Orthopedics
University of Colorado School of Medicine
Aurora, CO, United States

Robin West, MD
Chairman
Sports Medicine
Inova Health System
Fairfax, VA, United States

Associate Professor
Department of Orthopaedics
Georgetown Univeristy Medical Center
Washington, DC, United States

Head Team Physician
Washington Redskins
Ashburn, VA, United States

Lead Team Physician
Washington Nationals
Washington, DC, United States

Melissa N. Womble, PhD
Director, Neuropsychologist
Inova Sports Medicine
Inova Medical Group
Fairfax, VA, United States

Preface

Anterior cruciate ligament (ACL) injuries continue to be on the rise as younger population of both males and females increase their participation in youth, high-school, and collegiate sports. The largest increase has been seen in females; therefore, we wanted to focus on the impact, approach, and considerations of ACL surgery in the female athlete.

ACL Injuries in Female Athletes is meant to be an up-to-date reference that begins with the female ACL epidemic, discusses differences with respect to gender, and is one of the first of its kind to discuss the psychologic impact of and concerns with ACL injuries. The book takes the reader through the ACL epidemic, ACL biomechanics and anatomy, ACL graft choices, and biological healing after ACL surgery. It then adds topics on special considerations in the pediatric population as well as revision ACL surgery and strategies. Finally, the book focuses on the biological augmentation of ACL and rehabilitation and return to play following reconstruction and concludes with an in-depth look at the psychology of return to play following ACL reconstruction.

We are happy to present this collection of topics to our readers and its focus on the female athlete. We feel it represents a first of its kind compilation of the subject matter based on gender. As parents of youth female soccer players ourselves, this topic also resonates with us and our practices. We would also be remiss in acknowledging our many mentors, many of whom have also contributed to this body of work. We hope that you as the reader enjoy and find the book as a beneficial resource to add to your practice.

Robin West, MD
Brandon Bryant, BS, MD

Contents

CHAPTER 1

Anterior Cruciate Ligament Ruptures in the Female Athlete: An Injury Epidemic

MIGUEL A. PELTON, MD • EDWARD S. CHANG, MD

INTRODUCTION

Each year in the United States, approximately 250,000 anterior cruciate ligament (ACL) injuries occur. Mall et al.[1] reported an increase in ACL reconstruction from 32.94 per 100,000 person-years in 1994 to 43.48 per 100,000 person-years in 2006. This is likely attributed to both an increase in sports participation and a heightened awareness of the injury.

Females have consistently been shown to be more at risk for these injuries in a disproportionate manner, with a four- to six-fold increased risk of rupture.[2,3] One recent epidemiologic study assessed the trends of ACL injuries from 2002 to 2014 and the subsequent reconstruction procedures and found that the rates of ACL reconstruction per 100,000 person-years rose by 22%, i.e., from 61.4 in 2002 to 74.6 in 2014. During this period, females experienced a more rapid increase in reconstruction rate than males (34% vs. 13%, $P<.01$).[4] The often cited reasons for this increased risk of injury in female athletes include decreased neuromuscular control, smaller notch width, increased Q angles, and genetic and hormonal effects on type I collagen tissue.[5]

Epidemiologic studies have elucidated current and past trends with certain female sports and ACL injuries. Disproportionately affected sports include activities in which pivoting and cutting forces further strain an already "at-risk" ligament. Such sports include soccer, field hockey, volleyball, and gymnastics. This chapter evaluates the latest literature on epidemiologic trends of ACL injuries in female athletes. It will touch on the pathophysiology but will mostly focus on the most commonly affected sports and activities further stratified by age ranges. Lastly, the role of prevention programs in decreasing ACL injury rates in the female patient will be assessed.

PATHOPHYSIOLOGY

A noncontact pivoting moment on a flexed knee has been thought of as the main reason for an ACL rupture. This most commonly occurs while landing from a jump, sudden change of direction, or deceleration. Valgus collapse at the knee, decreased knee flexion angles (<30 degrees), and increased hip internal rotation are often reported during ACL injuries. Biomechanical studies have further shown the ACL to be under greater stress at this position[6] (Fig. 1.1).

A kinematic study assessed the peak cartilage pressures during landing from a drop vertical jump in young female athletes who went onto to develop ACL injury.[6] This group was compared with a group of females without subsequent ACL injury who performed the same kinematic testing, and it was found that the highest ACL strains occurred in the combined knee abduction/anterior tibial translation condition in the group that had a baseline knee abduction angle of 5 degrees. These injuries subsequently correlated to the bone bruise patterns noted on the lateral femoral condyle and posterolateral proximal tibia, likely from the valgus collapse.

Another study analyzed 205 female athletes in high-risk sports (soccer, volleyball, and basketball) and found that knee abduction angles of 8 degrees or higher, increased abduction/valgus moments, and increased ground reaction forces all increased the risk of ACL injuries.[7]

Multiple investigators have explored the details of the mechanism for failure.[7,8] Although certain anatomic factors in females (small notch width, increased Q angle, increased posterior tibial slope) have been associated with increased risk of injury, much of the recent interest and research has been on the biomechanical and neuromuscular factors related to ACL injury in females.

Four theories have been introduced to describe the biomechanics and neuromuscular role in ACL injury: the ligament dominance theory, the trunk dominance theory, the quadriceps dominance theory, and the leg dominance theory[8] (Table 1.1).

The ligament dominance theory suggests that female athletes at high risk perform athletic maneuvers with excessive knee valgus, hip adduction, and hip internal rotation. The trunk dominance theory suggests that poor

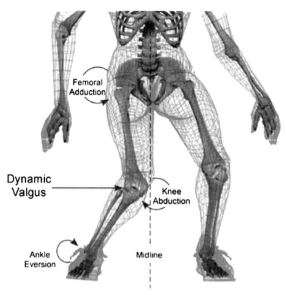

FIG. 1.1 Proposed mechanism for anterior cruciate ligament (ACL) injuries in females. Combination of motions and rotations at all three lower extremity joints, potentially including hip adduction and internal rotation, knee abduction, tibial external rotation and anterior translation, and ankle eversion. (Reprinted from Hewett TE, Myer GD, Ford KR. Anterior cruciate ligament injuries in female athletes: part 1, mechanisms and risk factors. *Am J Sports Med*. 2006;34(2):299–311.)

TABLE 1.1
ACL Tear Risk Factors in Female Athletes

Risk Factor	Proposed Mechanism
Genetics[11]	*ACAN* (aggrecan): Aggregating proteoglycan that plays a critical role in mediating chondrocyte-chondrocyte and chondrocyte-matrix interactions. Resists compression and shear forces by attracting water molecules into tissue spaces. • ACAN upregulation can potentially result in increased ACAN secretion in the ACL and consequently a disproportionate increase of ACAN relative to the total composition of the tissue • **increased ACAN secretion can lead to compositional changes in females and increased risk for ACL rupture** COL5A1 encodes for the α1 chain of type V collagen, which is a minor fibrillar collagen found in ligaments and tendons, as well as other tissues. **COL5A1 BstUI RFLP may be underrepresented in female participants with ACL ruptures** *FMOD* (fibromodulin): Encodes the protein fibromodulin. This is found in a variety of musculoskeletal tissues (including ligaments), controls collagen fibril formation, and inhibits the growth of types I and II collagen fibrils in vitro. • increased expression of fibromodulin results in delayed collagen fibril formation and thinner fibrils • **upregulation of FMOD found in ACL tissue from female participants compared with male participants may indicate an overall inhibition of collagen fibrillogenesis** *WISP* (WNT1 inducible signaling pathway protein 2): Multifunctional protein that is secreted by many other cell types and is involved in extracellular matrix regulation. • **downregulation of WISP2 in females may negatively affect cellular proliferation and growth, extracellular matrix control and deposition, and other factors determining ligament composition and structure**
Age[11–14]	• Age and gender were identified as risk factors for contralateral ACL reconstruction. • Youngest age group (13–15 years) showed an increased risk of contralateral ACL surgery compared with the reference (36–49 years) age group[11] • Higher activity level of younger patients, both pre- and postoperatively. Eagerness to return to competitive sport as soon as possible could also be a contributing factor.

TABLE 1.1 ACL Tear Risk Factors in Female Athletes—cont'd	
Risk Factor	**Proposed Mechanism**
Sport type[17]	Relative risk was highest in basketball (3.80; 95% CI, 2.53–5.85) and soccer (3.67; 95% CI, 2.61–5.27). • female soccer had the highest rate of injury per exposure • **highest injury rates were observed in soccer, football, basketball, and lacrosse, while volleyball had the lowest injury rate among female sports and baseball**[42–44]
Landing biomechanics[6–8]	**Quadriceps dominance**: Excessive relative quadriceps forces or reduced hamstring recruitment place the ACL at high risk for injury. **Leg dominance**: Large leg-to-leg asymmetries predispose athletes to injury. **Trunk dominance**: Poor trunk control during athletic maneuvers leads to increased risk for ACL injury. **Ligament dominance**: Female athletes at high risk perform athletic maneuvers with excessive knee valgus, hip adduction, and hip internal rotation. **Most prevalent group for ACL injuries were a combination of deficits.**
Anatomy/hormonal[7,45–47]	**Larger Q angle:** Leads to a more laterally directed pull of the quadriceps at the knee, which may place the ACL in a position in which it is more prone to rupture.[7] **Smaller notch width**[28]: Statistically significant difference was found between the sex of the athlete and notch width indices or rate of ACL tears. The notch width index may not be the ideal measure because as subjects grow taller, the femoral condylar width increases disproportionately compared with the intercondylar notch width. **Increased posterior tibial slope:** An increased posterior tibial slope increases tibial translation and ACL strain. **Estrogen:** Increased estrogen (ovulatory) phase associated with negative fibroblast proliferation and increases ACL laxity, although this does not correlate with increased ACL tear.

ACL, anterior cruciate ligament.

trunk and core control during athletic maneuvers leads to increased risk for ACL injury. The quadriceps dominance theory suggests that excessive relative quadriceps forces or reduced hamstring recruitment places the ACL at high risk for injury. Lastly, the leg dominance theory suggests that large leg-to-leg asymmetries predispose athletes to injury.[8]

While each of these theories has studies supporting them, it is likely that a combination of these biomechanical "deficits" will place the female athlete at a high risk for ACL injury.

Pappas et al. used lower extremity 3D kinematic and kinetic analysis to assess 721 high-school female athletes performing a cutting task. They found that 40% of the subjects demonstrated no biomechanical deficits and were at low risk for ACL injury.[8] In the other group, the authors noted that 77% exhibited a combination of deficits and only 24% was classified as having a single deficit. This study and other such studies demonstrated the potentially modifiable risk factors for ACL injury that have led to research in the development of neuromuscular training (NMT) programs.

GENETIC AND HORMONAL RISK FACTORS
There has been considerable interest in establishing a genetic link for ACL injuries in at-risk females. COL5A1

is a gene that encodes for the α1 chain of type I collagen. It has been speculated that downregulation of this gene may be responsible for ACL injuries in females. Posthumus and colleagues[45] compared 129 white participants (38 women) with surgically diagnosed ACL ruptures and 216 physically active control participants (84 women) without any history of ACL injury. They found that the COL5A1 genotype in the female participants was significantly underrepresented in the ACL rupture group compared with the controls. John et al. [46] characterized the amalgamation of genetic studies in their systematic review. The included articles looked at 20 specific genetic polymorphisms and found genetic associations with ACL injury, including COL3A1, COL12A1, and COL1A1. Johnson et al.[47] conducted a study to compare gene expression and structural features in torn ACL tissue obtained intraoperatively from young female and male athletes during surgical ACL reconstruction. The authors further identified three genes of interest by performing reverse transcription quantitative polymerase chain reaction: *ACAN* (aggrecan), *FMOD* (fibromodulin), and *WISP2* (WNT1 inducible signaling pathway protein 2). They found that *ACAN* and *FMOD* were upregulated in female vs. male subjects, whereas *WISP2* was downregulated. These genotypic studies further support the theory that females are potentially more at risk for ACL injuries. More investigations, however, are needed to further support the phenotypic expression of these polymorphisms.

There also has been research potentially correlating hormonal differences between sexes as a potential risk factor for ACL injuries in women. Liu et al.[49] showed that estrogen and progesterone receptors were found in the cells of the ligament, including the fibroblasts and synoviocytes. Furthermore, Yu et al.[50] found that estrogen had a negative effect on fibroblast proliferation and collagen synthesis.

Multiple studies were then performed to evaluate whether there was greater risk of ACL injuries based on the ovulatory phase.[48] Zazulak et al.[51] performed a systematic review and found that although ACL laxity was greater in the ovulatory phase (high estrogen), injuries were found to be higher in the follicular phase (low estrogen).

AGE AND ANTERIOR CRUCIATE LIGAMENT INJURIES IN FEMALES

With the increasing rates of participation in high-risk sports at an earlier age, the correlation between age and ACL injury was investigated.[9] Several studies have summarized the rates of ACL injuries in younger patients, with some even stratifying outcomes based on gender. Webster and Feller[10] sought to investigate a large cohort of patients at 1 year following ACL reconstruction to determine if range of motion, knee laxity, objective performance measures, and validated

outcome scores differed according to gender, age; and sport participation status. They showed that men, following ACL reconstruction, had less knee laxity, greater limb symmetry, and higher International Knee Documentation Committee scores than women. All outcomes measures showed higher scores and reduced deficits in younger patients. This was most true for patients in the very youngest group (<16 years old) when compared with the oldest group (>45 years old). Another study out of the Swedish registry found that females had a 33.7% greater risk of contralateral ACL surgery. It also found that the youngest age group (13–15 years, 16.7%) showed an increased risk of contralateral ACL surgery compared with the reference (36–49 years, 8.6%) age group.[11] These and other studies seem to demonstrate that younger patients and females are at more increased risk for contralateral ACL injuries and the subsequent need for contralateral ACL reconstruction.[12–14]

SPORTS-SPECIFIC ANTERIOR CRUCIATE LIGAMENT EPIDEMIOLOGY (TABLE 1.2)
Soccer

Soccer is the most commonly played sport worldwide with an estimated 240 million active players.[15] Most injuries occur in the lower extremity and more specifically at the knee joint.[16] Many epidemiologic studies have been performed to investigate the trends of soccer injuries worldwide. Female athletes appear to have increased ACL injury rates, increased rates of ACL reconstruction procedures, and decreased return to preinjury

TABLE 1.2
Anterior Cruciate Ligament Female Incidence by Sport

References	Sport	Injury Rate (Per exposures or Relative Risk)
Gornitzky et al.[17]	Soccer	RR 3.67 (per exposure) IR 0.148 (per 1000 exposures)
Agel et al.[25]	Basketball	0.16 (per 1000 exposures)
Renstrom et al.[32]	Volleyball	0.09 (per 1000 athlete exposures)
Verhagen et al.[33]	Volleyball	2.6 (per 1000 exposure hours)
Hootman et al.[28]	Softball	4.3 (per 1000 athlete exposures)
Swenson et al.[36]	Gymnastics	4.23 (per 10,000 athlete exposures)
Mountcastle et al.[37]	Gymnastics	0.24 (per 1000 athlete exposures)
Agel et al.[38]	Gymnastics	0.24 (per 1000 athlete exposures)
Agel et al.[38]	Field hockey	0.11 (per 1000 athlete exposures)
Beynnon et al.[40]	Field hockey	0.038 and 0.048 per 1000 person-days for women's (college) field hockey and girls' (high school) field hockey, respectively

IR, injury rate; *RR*, relative risk.

participation status (Table 1.1). A recent meta-analysis of a total of 700 ACL injuries in 11,239,029 exposures in high-school athletes found that females had a higher rate of injury per exposure (relative risk, 1.57).[17] In these females, relative risk was highest in basketball (3.80) and soccer (3.67). Boys' football had the highest number of ACL injuries at 273 of the 700 total ACL injuries, whereas girls' soccer had the highest injury rate per 1000 exposures of 0.148.

In girls' sports the highest injury risks per season were observed in soccer (1.11%), basketball (0.88%), and lacrosse (0.53%). The Multicenter Orthopaedic Outcomes Network (MOON) group is an ongoing multicenter prospective cohort that evaluates both short- and long-term outcomes following ACL reconstruction.[18] Based on multivariate analysis, older patients and females were less likely to return to soccer. Additionally, females were significantly more likely to have future ACL surgery (20% vs. 5.5%) than men.

Similarly, a Swedish questionnaire of 300 soccer players found that only 28% of male and female soccer players continued to play soccer 3 years after ACL injury.[19] At 7 years' follow-up of patients undergoing ACL reconstruction, it was found that only 26% of men and 12% of women were still playing. The range of incidence of ACL injury is from 0.06 to 10 per 1000 game hours in the reported literature.[20] Additionally, female soccer players have a two- to three-fold increased risk for ACL injury when compared with their male counterparts.[15,21,22]

Basketball

Female basketball players have a 5.3-times higher relative risk of valgus collapse during ACL injury than male basketball players.[23] It has also been shown that next to soccer, basketball results in the second highest incidence of ACL injuries. During the 2007–08 academic year, an estimated 556,269 boys and 456,967 girls participated in this sport.[24] It was found that knee ligament injuries (47%) were the most common injuries seen in girls and that females had a much higher proportion of knee injuries than males (injury proportion ratio, 1.71). Agel and colleagues[25] reported a significant difference in the rate of noncontact ACL ruptures over a 13-year period (1990–2002) between female and male collegiate basketball players (0.16 and 0.04 injuries per 1000 exposures respectively, $P<.01$). Another study investigated sex-specific differences in the types of injuries sustained by basketball players.[26] It was found that in the 10- to 19-year-old age group the proportion of ACL injuries was higher in female than in male players (45.9% vs. 22.1%).

SOFTBALL

USA Softball registers over 245,000 softball teams, comprising more than 3.5 million players (among them, there are more than 83,000 youth girls' fast-pitch teams, with over 1.2 million girls).[27] While multiple studies have demonstrated that ACL injuries occur more often in soccer and basketball, females continue to be at higher risk of ACL injury than their male counterparts.[28,29] Stanley and colleagues[27] analyzed knee ligamentous injury and athlete-exposure data from the National Athletic Treatment, Injury and Outcomes Network (NATION) and the National Collegiate Athletic Association (NCAA) Injury Surveillance Program (ISP) during the 2009–10 to 2013–14 academic years. The authors found that ACL injury rates in females were higher at both the collegiate and high-school levels. Additionally, at the collegiate level the highest ACL injury incidence rate ratios (IRRs) comparing female to male athletes was reported in softball/baseball [IRR, 6.61; 95% confidence interval (CI), 1.48–29.55].

VOLLEYBALL

Over a 5-year period, one epidemiologic study demonstrated that volleyball consisted of 8.8% of all ACL injuries in high-school females.[29] Sole and colleagues[31] found that over a 4–year period, the knee was the most commonly injured body region in female collegiate volleyball NCAA division I athletes. One Swedish registry study found that over a period of 16 years of 5000 ACL injuries, female volleyball players made up to 2.0% of the injuries (0.09 injury rate per 1000 athlete exposures).[32] Verhagen et al.[33] reported an overall injury rate of 2.6 injuries/1000 h, with 5% of all volleyball injuries being acute knee injuries. Agel et al.[38] noted 3.7% of all volleyball-related injuries were related to the ACL. Although volleyball ACL injuries represent a minority of the acute knee injuries, significant research is underway to reduce the rates in this popular sport.[30,34,35]

GYMNASTICS

Swenson and colleagues[36] studied a cohort of athletes in multiple sports from 2005 to 2011. They found that the injury rates for females in gymnastics were 4.23 per 10,000 athlete exposures. Mountcastle et al.[37] assessed ACL injuries at the US Military Academy at West Point from 1994 to 2003 and found that women had a significantly increased rate of ACL injury then men in gymnastics (0.24 and 0.04 per 1000 exposures, $P<.001$).

Interestingly, Agel et al.[38] showed that collegiate female gymnasts showed a significant decrease in incidence of ACL injuries between 2004 and 2013. This resulted in a 2.8% ACL injury rate of all the injuries in the 15 NCAA sports and 0.24 injury rate per 1000 athlete exposures. The authors did not mention as to why this decreased trend was observed; however, injury prevention programs and identification of ACL risk factor studies may have contributed to the decrease during this time frame.

FIELD HOCKEY

Given the nature of ball handling, field players assume a crouched position with high degrees of both trunk and knee flexion. These actions can lead to a decreased risk for ACL injury compared with lacrosse.[39] Agel and colleagues[38] found an overall ACL injury rate of 0.11 per 1000 athlete exposures in their pooled date from 2004 to 2013. Their data demonstrates a 57% increase in overall injury rate between the original 15-year and subsequent 9-year study period.[25] Beynnon et al.[40] assessed first-time noncontact ACL injury rates over a period of 4 years from pooled data of 8 colleges and 18 high schools across 7 sports. They found overall low injury rates of 0.038 and 0.048 per 1000 person-days for women's (college) field hockey and girls' (high school) field hockey, respectively.

EFFECTS OF NEUROMUSCULAR TRAINING PROGRAMS ON ANTERIOR CRUCIATE LIGAMENT INJURY EPIDEMIOLOGY

Much insight and research is seeking ways to reduce the rates of ACL injuries in females.[41] The effects of NMT on female athletes is becoming popular in the literature.[42] These studies evaluate whether training of female athletes to improve biomechanical deficits of elevated knee abduction, limited knee flexion, asymmetric landing patterns, higher ground reaction force, and poor trunk control can decrease rates of ACL injuries.[43] A systematic review assessed the effects of NMT on ACL injuries in females based on duration, frequency, and volume of NMT.[44] A total of 14 studies were included that showed greater ACL injury reduction in female athletes who were in the long NMT duration group [odds ratio (OR), 0.35; 95% CI, 0.23, 0.53; $P = .001$] than those in the short NMT duration group (OR, 0.61; 95% CI, 0.41, 0.90; $P = .013$). Additionally, when they compared single NMT frequency (only one session per week during season) with multi-NMT frequency (two or more sessions per week), they found a greater ACL injury reduction in the latter (OR, 0.35; 95% CI, 0.23, 0.53; $P = .001$) than in the former (OR, 0.62; 95%

CI, 0.41, 0.94; $P = .024$). Lastly, high-volume (greater 30 min) and moderate-volume (15–30 min) NMT sessions showed increased reduction in ACL injury rates over low-volume NMT sessions.

CONCLUSION

As sports participation continues to increase, especially among the youth, ACL injuries remain a significant concern for female athletes. Most epidemiologic studies estimate that female athletes are two to eight times more likely to sustain an ACL injury than male athletes. Furthermore, females are at greater risk to rupture the contralateral ACL following returning to play from an ACL injury. Several sports have intrinsic risk factors to create the potential for injuries in the at-risk knee. Certain anatomic and neuromuscular differences may contribute to the higher rates seen in females. Multiple neuromuscular and proprioceptive protocols have been designed and early studies are promising, showing reduced incidence of ACL injury following completion of the program. Further research is necessary to identify the main risk factors for ACL injuries in female athletes and, just as important, correct the modifiable factors.

REFERENCES

1. Mall NA, et al. Incidence and trends of anterior cruciate ligament reconstruction in the United States. *Am J Sports Med.* 2014;42(10):2363–2370.
2. Arendt EA, Agel J, Dick R. Anterior cruciate ligament injury patterns among collegiate men and women. *J Athl Train.* 1999;34(2):86–92.
3. Marquez G, et al. Sex differences in kinetic and neuromuscular control during jumping and landing. *J Musculoskelet Neuronal Interact.* 2017;17(1):409–416.
4. Herzog MM, et al. Incidence of anterior cruciate ligament reconstruction among adolescent females in the United States, 2002 through 2014. *JAMA Pediatr.* 2017;171(8):808–810.
5. Herzberg SD, et al. The effect of menstrual cycle and contraceptives on ACL injuries and laxity: a systematic review and meta-analysis. *Orthop J Sports Med.* 2017;5(7):2325967117718781.
6. Quatman CE, et al. Cartilage pressure distributions provide a footprint to define female anterior cruciate ligament injury mechanisms. *Am J Sports Med.* 2011;39(8):1706–1713.
7. Hewett TE, et al. Biomechanical measures of neuromuscular control and valgus loading of the knee predict anterior cruciate ligament injury risk in female athletes: a prospective study. *Am J Sports Med.* 2005;33(4):492–501.
8. Pappas E, et al. Biomechanical deficit profiles associated with ACL injury risk in female athletes. *Med Sci Sports Exerc.* 2016;48(1):107–113.

9. Shaw L, Finch CF. Trends in pediatric and adolescent anterior cruciate ligament injuries in Victoria, Australia 2005-2015. *Int J Environ Res Public Health.* 2017;14(6).

10. Webster KE, Feller JA. Younger patients and men achieve higher outcome scores than older patients and women after anterior cruciate ligament reconstruction. *Clin Orthop Relat Res.* 2017 Oct;475(10):2472–2480. doi: 10.1007/s11999-017-5418-2.

11. Snaebjornsson T, et al. Adolescents and female patients are at increased risk for contralateral anterior cruciate ligament reconstruction: a cohort study from the Swedish National Knee Ligament Register based on 17,682 patients. *Knee Surg Sports Traumatol Arthrosc.* 2017 Dec;25(12):3938–3944. doi: 10.1007/s00167-017-4517-7. Epub 2017 Mar 15.

12. Shelbourne KD, Gray T, Haro M. Incidence of subsequent injury to either knee within 5 years after anterior cruciate ligament reconstruction with patellar tendon autograft. *Am J Sports Med.* 2009;37(2):246–251.

13. Mohtadi N, et al. Reruptures, reinjuries, and revisions at a minimum 2-year follow-up: a randomized clinical trial comparing 3 graft types for ACL reconstruction. *Clin J Sport Med.* 2016;26(2):96–107.

14. Webster KE, et al. Younger patients are at increased risk for graft rupture and contralateral injury after anterior cruciate ligament reconstruction. *Am J Sports Med.* 2014;42(3):641–647.

15. Waldén M, et al. The epidemiology of anterior cruciate ligament injury in football (soccer): a review of the literature from a gender-related perspective. *Knee Surg. Sports Traumatol Arthrosc.* 2011;19(1):3–10.

16. Chomiak J, et al. Severe injuries in football players. Influencing factors. *Am J Sports Med.* 2000;28(suppl 5):S58–S68.

17. Gornitzky AL, et al. Sport-specific yearly risk and incidence of anterior cruciate ligament tears in high school athletes. *Am J Sports Med.* 2016;44(10):2716–2723.

18. Brophy RH, et al. Return to play and future ACL injury risk after ACL reconstruction in soccer athletes from the multicenter orthopaedic outcomes Network (MOON) group. *Am J Sports Med.* 2012;40(11):2517–2522.

19. Roos H, et al. Soccer after anterior cruciate ligament injury–an incompatible combination? A national survey of incidence and risk factors and a 7-year follow-up of 310 players. *Acta Orthop Scand.* 1995;66(2):107–112.

20. Rochcongar P, et al. Ruptures of the anterior cruciate ligament in soccer. *Int J Sports Med.* 2009;30(5):372–378.

21. Prodromos CC, et al. A meta-analysis of the incidence of anterior cruciate ligament tears as a function of gender, sport, and a knee injury-reduction regimen. *Arthroscopy.* 2007;23(12):1320–1325.e6.

22. Brophy RH, et al. Defending puts the anterior cruciate ligament at risk during soccer: a gender-based analysis. *Sports Health.* 2015;7(3):244–249.

23. Krosshaug T, et al. Mechanisms of anterior cruciate ligament injury in basketball: video analysis of 39 cases. *Am J Sports Med.* 2007;35(3):359–367.

24. Borowski LA, et al. The epidemiology of US high school basketball injuries, 2005-2007. *Am J Sports Med.* 2008;36(12):2328–2335.

25. Agel J, Arendt EA, Bershadsky B. Anterior cruciate ligament injury in national collegiate athletic association basketball and soccer: a 13-year review. *Am J Sports Med.* 2005;33(4):524–530.

26. Ito E, et al. Sex-specific differences in injury types among basketball players. *Open Access J Sports Med.* 2015;6:1–6.

27. Stanley LE, et al. Sex differences in the incidence of anterior cruciate ligament, medial collateral ligament, and meniscal injuries in collegiate and high school sports. *Am J Sports Med.* 2016;44(6):1565–1572.

28. Hootman JM, Dick R, Agel J. Epidemiology of collegiate injuries for 15 sports: summary and recommendations for injury prevention initiatives. *J Athl Train.* 2007;42(2):311–319.

29. Joseph AM, et al. A multisport epidemiologic comparison of anterior cruciate ligament injuries in high school athletics. *J Athl Train.* 2013;48(6):810–817.

30. Bahr R, Bahr IA. Incidence of acute volleyball injuries: a prospective cohort study of injury mechanisms and risk factors. *Scand J Med Sci Sports.* 1997;7(3):166–171.

31. Sole C, Kavanaugh A, Stone M. Injuries in collegiate Women's volleyball: a four-year retrospective analysis. *Sports.* 2017;5(2):26.

32. Renstrom P, et al. Non-contact ACL injuries in female athletes: an International Olympic Committee current concepts statement. *Br J Sports Med.* 2008;42(6):394–412.

33. Verhagen EALM, et al. A one season prospective cohort study of volleyball injuries. *Br J Sports Med.* 2004;38(4):477–481.

34. Reeser JC, et al. Strategies for the prevention of volleyball related injuries. *Br J Sports Med.* 2006;40(7):594–600.

35. Ferretti A, et al. Knee ligament injuries in volleyball players. *Am J Sports Med.* 1992;20(2):203–207.

36. Swenson DM, et al. Epidemiology of knee injuries among US high school athletes, 2005/06–2010/11. *Med Sci Sports Exerc.* 2013;45(3):462–469.

37. Mountcastle SB, et al. Gender differences in anterior cruciate ligament injury vary with activity: epidemiology of anterior cruciate ligament injuries in a young, athletic population. *Am J Sports Med.* 2007;35(10):1635–1642.

38. Agel J, Rockwood T, Klossner D. Collegiate ACL injury rates across 15 sports: national collegiate athletic association injury surveillance system data update (2004-2005 through 2012-2013). *Clin J Sport Med.* 2016;26(6):518–523.

39. Braun HJ, et al. Differences in ACL biomechanical risk factors between field hockey and lacrosse female athletes. *Knee Surg Sports Traumatol Arthrosc.* 2015;23(4):1065–1070.

40. Beynnon BD, et al. The effects of level of competition, sport, and sex on the incidence of first-time noncontact anterior cruciate ligament injury. *Am J Sports Med.* 2014;42(8):1806–1812.

41. Grimm NL, et al. Anterior cruciate ligament and knee injury prevention programs for soccer players. *Am J Sports Med.* 2015;43(8):2049–2056.

42. Emery CA, et al. Neuromuscular training injury prevention strategies in youth sport: a systematic review and meta-analysis. *Br J Sports Med.* 2015;49(13):865–870.

43. Sugimoto D, et al. Critical components of neuromuscular training to reduce ACL injury risk in female athletes: meta-regression analysis. *Br J Sports Med.* 2016 Oct;50(20):1259–1266. doi: 10.1136/bjsports-2015-095596. Epub 2016 Jun 1.

44. Sugimoto D, et al. Dosage effects of neuromuscular training intervention to reduce anterior cruciate ligament injuries in female athletes: meta-and sub-group analyses. Auckland, N.Z. *Sports Med.* 2014;44(4):551–562.

45. Posthumus M, et al. The COL5I1 gene is associated with increased risk of anterior cruciate ligament ruptures in female participants. *Am J Sports Med.* 2009;37(11):2234–2240.

46. John R, et al. Is there a genetic predisposition to anterior cruciate ligament tear? A systematic review. *Am J Sports Med.* 2016;44(12):3262–3269.

47. Johnson JS, et al. Gene expression differences between ruptured anterior cruciate ligaments in young male and female subjects. *J Bone Joint Surg Am.* 2015;97(1):71–79.

48. Sutton KM, et al. Anterior cruciate ligament rupture: differences between males and females. *J Am Acad Orthop Surg.* 2013;21(1):41–50.

49. Liu SH, et al. Primary immunolocalization of estrogen and progesterone target cells in the human anterior cruciate ligament. *J Orthop Res.* 1996;14(4):526–533.

50. Yu WD, et al. Combined effects of estrogen and progesterone on the anterior cruciate ligament. *Clin Orthop Relat Res.* 2001;383:268–281.

51. Zazulak BT, et al. The effects of the menstrual cycle on anterior knee laxity: a systematic review. 2006;36(10):847–862.

CHAPTER 2

Epidemiology

PATRICK WAKEFIELD JOYNER, MD, MS • BRYAN L. GOLDSTEIN, BA

There are an estimated 200,000 anterior cruciate ligament (ACL) injuries reported in the United States each year, many of which occur due to sports injuries.[1,2] Female athletes are anywhere from two to nine times more likely to sustain a noncontact ACL injury than their male counterparts, with the highest rate of incidence occurring in the 15- to 40-year-old age range.[3–5]

A noncontact injury is where one athlete sustains damage during an awkward movement without direct contact with another athlete. High-risk movement for noncontact injuries include jumping, cutting, pivoting, and stopping or decelerating suddenly, which are commonly associated with sports such as soccer, basketball, football, and gymnastics.[4,6] According to a study by Prodromos et al.,[6] female athletes who participate in year-round soccer and basketball have an approximate 5% ACL tear rate. The National Collegiate Athletic Association (NCAA) reports that lower-extremity injuries accounted for approximately 53% across both the sexes between 1988–89 and 2003–04 athletic seasons, with 4800 documented ACL injuries, 1515 of which occurred in female athletes (Fig. 2.1).[7]

However, over the years, female participation in collegiate-level organized sports has increased by approximately 80%, which has led to an increase in ACL injury rates as well.[7] Among female athletes at the high-school level, there is an estimated 20,000–80,000 ACL injuries per year.[8]

With the consistent upward trend incidence of ACL injury in female athletes, the number of ACL reconstructions performed each year has also increased. Between 1994 and 2006, the number of ACL reconstructions performed on females in the United States increased from a rate of 20.5 per 100,000 capita to a rate of 36.2 per 100,000 capita.[9] The rate of successful outcomes following initial ACL reconstruction is reported to range from 75% to 97%.[2]

There are multiple hypotheses regarding the reason female athletes are at a higher risk of sustaining ACL injuries. The leading hypotheses have to do with sex-based anatomic differences, hormone cycling, and neuromuscular deficits in females.[10] Some research has suggested that a wider pelvis in females causes an increase in the valgus angle

between the femur's long axis and the tibia. Further testing of this hypothesis has provided mixed results. Some of the research shows support for increased risk of ACL injury due to this increased valgus angle, whereas other results have demonstrated no correlation. Another anatomic hypothesis suggests differences in femoral notch size relative to the size of the ACL. However, subsequent research has not shown any difference in femoral notch size between males and females.[10]

The hormonal hypothesis suggests that cycling of female sex hormones, beginning at puberty and continuing to maturity, leads to decreased ligament strength in females.[2,10] Research has been conducted on female athletes across the menstrual cycle phases with mixed results. There is evidence to support a generalized increase in joint flexibility and ligament laxity in females, and a decrease in males, with chronologic age and maturation stage and may contribute to increased ACL injury rate following puberty.[2] The neuromuscular theory suggests the dynamic muscular restraints to joint loads fail to properly compensate for the high dynamic load on the knee joint and protect the ACL.[10] Power, strength, and coordination have been shown to increase with chronologic age and maturity in males but this has not been observed in females.[10]

ANATOMY

The ACL is a ligament that functions to prevent hyperextension of the tibia, excessive internal rotation of the tibia, and anterior shifting of the tibia from underneath the femur; it is tight during extension and loose during flexion.[11] The ACL originates on the medial anterior aspect of the tibial plateau and runs superiorly, laterally, and posteriorly to the point of insertion on the medial aspect of the lateral femoral condyle. On the macroscopic level, the ACL is composed of two main bundles: the anteromedial (AM) and posterolateral (PL) bundles (Fig. 2.2).[11,12] The bundles are named from their respective insertion points on the anterior intercondylar area of the tibia. These two bundles supply roughly 85% of

ACL Injuries in Female Athletes. https://doi.org/10.1016/B978-0-323-54839-7.00002-6

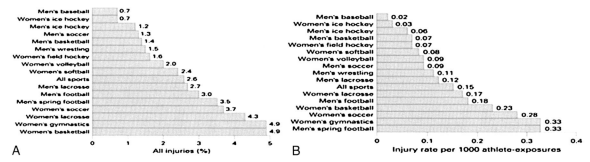

FIG. 2.1 Occurrence of anterior cruciate ligament (ACL) injury expressed as **(A)** percentage of all injuries and **(B)** the rate per 1000 exposures (games and practices combined, 1988–89 through 2003–04).[3]

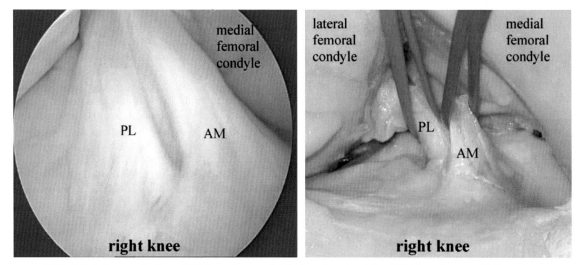

FIG. 2.2 Arthroscopic view of **(A)** the anteromedial (AM) and posterolateral (PL) bundles and **(B)** the anterior aspect of a human cadaver knee.[12]

the total restraining for anterior translation of the knee joint.[11] The tensions of the two bundles contradict; the AM bundle is loose in extension and the PL bundle is tight.[13] The AM bundle becomes tight and the PL bundle becomes loose during flexion of the knee because of the more horizontal orientation of the ACL. The AM and PL bundle lengths are significantly different, with the AM bundle measuring on average around 36.9 mm in length and 5.1 mm in width and the PL bundle measuring on average 20.5 mm in length and 4.4 mm in width (based on sagittal views).[4] The AM bundle is representative of the overall length of the ACL.

At the microscopic level, the ACL can be divided into three zones: proximal, middle, and distal.[14] The proximal zone has a high content of round and ovoid

cells, along with some fusiform fibroblasts, type II collagen, and glycoproteins. The middle, or fusiform, zone is rich in fusiform and spindle-shaped fibroblasts. This zone also contains a high density of cartilage and fibrocartilage, elastic fibers, and oxytalan fibers. The function of the oxytalan fibers is to absorb modest stress from multiple directions, whereas the function of the elastic fibers is to absorb maximal stress.[14] The distal zone contains a high concentration of chondroblasts and ovoid fibroblasts.[14]

There are five genicular arteries: superomedial, superolateral, middle, inferomedial, and inferolateral, with the majority of the ACL being vascularized by the middle genicular artery (MGA).[14,15] The genicular arteries are branches of the popliteal artery, with the MGA originating at a right angle from its anterior aspect. The MGA branches once it has entered the joint space and is able to supply blood to the ACL of other nearby soft tissues via capillaries.

It has been demonstrated that the blood supply throughout the ACL is not evenly distributed, with the proximal section having a greater concentration of blood vessels.[14] The distal part of the ACL is vascularized by the inferior genicular arteries, in part, and is less vascularized than the other portions of the ACL.[14] There is also an avascular zone in the ACL at the anterior fibrocartilaginous area near the tibial insertion point.[14]

BIOMECHANICS

The stability of the knee is affected by ligamentous and neuromuscular restraints, which are categorized as passive and active, respectively. During common sports maneuvers, including landing, pivoting, and cutting, both the passive and active restraints are thought to play a role in the stabilization and protection of the knee joint. Differences between the knee joint biomechanics of female and male athletes have been observed that are considered to increase the risk of ACL injury in females.

ACL injuries have been observed to occur under high dynamic loads on the knee joint coupled with inadequate compensation by muscular restraints to protect the knee joint.[16] The various muscles of the leg work cooperatively to provide dynamic knee stabilization during pivoting and landing, especially the hamstrings and quadriceps muscles are observed to co-contract.[16]

When female athletes land they demonstrate greater knee extension, increased valgus pronation angles, as well as decreased knee and hip flexion. Decreased hip abduction during landing and cutting maneuvers are also common.[17,18] Jackson et al.[19] reported that before puberty, there is no difference observed in the biomechanics of the lower limb in males and females during landing maneuvers. However, after puberty, it has been observed that the increased bone length in the absence of neuromuscular adaptation in female athletes may lead to increased knee abduction moment (KAM) and thus increased ACL injury rates.[20] An increase in KAM is therefore a potential indicator for ACL injury risk.

According to Myer et al.,[16] female athletes who suffered ACL injury demonstrated a decreased hamstring strength and similar relative quadriceps strength when compared with uninjured male athletes. When low hamstring strength is coupled with a relatively high quadriceps strength, female athletes are at higher risk of ACL injury during sports maneuvers, such as those previously mentioned.

REFERENCES

1. Paterno MV, Rauh MJ, Schmitt LC, Ford KR, Hewett TE. Incidence of contralateral and ipsilateral anterior cruciate ligament (ACL) injury after primary ACL reconstruction and return to sport. Clinical journal of sport medicine. *Off J Can Acad Sport Med.* 2012;22(2):116–121. https://doi.org/10.1097/JSM.0b013e318246ef9e.
2. Kamath GV, Redfern JC, Greis PE, Burks RT. Revision anterior cruciate ligament reconstruction. *Am J Sports Med.* 2010;39(1):199–217. https://doi.org/10.1177/0363546510370929.
3. Myer GD, Ford KR, Paterno MV, Nick TG, Hewett TE. The effects of generalized joint laxity on risk of anterior cruciate ligament injury in young female athletes. *Am J Sports Med.* 2008;36(6):1073–1080. https://doi.org/10.1177/0363546507313572.
4. Voskanian NACL. Injury prevention in female athletes: review of the literature and practical considerations in implementing an ACL prevention program. *Curr Rev Musculoskelet Med.* 2013;6(2):158–163. https://doi.org/10.1007/s12178-013-9158-y.
5. Lind M, Menhert F, Pedersen AB. Incidence and outcome after revision anterior cruciate ligament reconstruction. *Am J Sports Med.* 2012;40(7):1551–1557. https://doi.org/10.1177/0363546512446000.
6. Prodromos CC, Han Y, Rogowski J, Joyce B, Shi K. A meta-analysis of the incidence of anterior cruciate ligament tears as a function of gender, sport, and a knee injury–reduction regimen. *Arthrosc J Arthrosc Relat Surg.* 2007;(12):23. https://doi.org/10.1016/j.arthro.2007.07.003.
7. Hootman JM, Dick R, Agel J. Epidemiology of collegiate injuries for 15 sports: summary and recommendations for injury prevention Initiatives. *J Athl Train.* 2007;42(2): 311–319.
8. Labella CR, Huxford MR, Grissom J, Kim K-Y, Peng J, Christoffel KK. Effect of neuromuscular warm-up on injuries in female soccer and basketball athletes in urban public high schools. *Arch Pediatr Adolesc Med.* 2011;165(11):1033. https://doi.org/10.1001/archpediatrics.2011.168.
9. Buller LT, Best MJ, Baraga MG, Kaplan LD. Trends in anterior cruciate ligament reconstruction in the United States. *Orthop J Sports Med.* 2015;3(1):2325967114563664 https://doi.org/10.1177/2325967114563664.
10. *Mechanisms. Mayo Clinic.* http://www.mayo.edu/research/labs/orthopedic-biomechanics/focus-areas/mechanisms?_ga=2.2696112.164327440.1511913218-1579963752.1511913218. Published February 27, 2017.

11. *Anterior Cruciate Ligament: Anatomy and Physiology.* Shpmissouriedu; 2018. Available at: https://shp.missouri.edu/vhct/case3505/anat_physio.htm.

12. Siebold R, Ellert T, Metz S, Metz J. Tibial insertions of the anteromedial and posterolateral bundles of the anterior cruciate ligament: morphometry, arthroscopic landmarks, and orientation model for bone tunnel placement. *Arthrosc J Arthrosc Relat Surg.* 2008;24(2):154–161. https://doi.org/10.1016/j.arthro.2007.08.006.

13. Zantop T, Petersen W, Sekiya J, Musahl V, Fu F. Anterior cruciate ligament anatomy and function relating to anatomical reconstruction. *Knee Surg Sports Traumatol Arthrosc.* 2006;14(10):982–992. https://doi.org/10.1007/s00167-006-0076-z.

14. Duthon V, Barea C, Abrassart S, Fasel J, Fritschy D, Ménétrey J. Anatomy of the anterior cruciate ligament. *Knee Surg Sports Traumatol Arthrosc.* 2005;14(3):204–213. https://doi.org/10.1007/s00167-005-0679-9.

15. Lazaro L, Cross M, Lorich D. Vascular anatomy of the patella: implications for total knee arthroplasty surgical approaches. *Knee.* 2014;21(3):655–660. https://doi.org/10.1016/j.knee.2014.03.005.

16. Myer GD, Ford KR, Foss KDB, Liu C, Nick TG, Hewett TE. The relationship of hamstrings and quadriceps strength to anterior cruciate ligament injury in female athletes. *Clin J Sport Med.* 2009;19(1):3–8. https://doi.org/10.1097/jsm.0b013e318190bddb.

17. Hopper AJ, Haff EE, Joyce C, Lloyd RS, Haff GG. Neuromuscular training improves lower extremity biomechanics associated with knee injury during landing in 11–13 Year old female netball athletes: a randomized control study. *Front Physiol.* 2017;8:883. https://doi.org/10.3389/fphys.2017.00883.

18. Holden SCA, Boreham C, Delahunt E. Sex differences in landing biomechanics and postural stability during adolescence: a systematic review with meta-analyses. *Sports Med.* 2015;46(2):241–253. https://doi.org/10.1007/s40279-015-0416-6.

19. Jackson KR, Garrison JC, Ingersoll CD, Hertel J. Similarity of hip and knee kinematics and kinetics among prepubescent boys and girls during a drop vertical jump landing. *Athl Train Sports Health Care.* 2010;2(2):74–80. https://doi.org/10.3928/19425864-20100226-07.

20. Hewett TE, Myer GD, Kiefer AW, Ford KR. Longitudinal increases in knee abduction moments in females during adolescent growth. *Med Sci Sports Exerc.* 2015;47(12):2579–2585. https://doi.org/10.1249/MSS.0000000000000700.

FURTHER READING

1. Cohen S, VanBeek C, Starman J, Armfield D, Irrgang J, Fu F. MRI measurement of the 2 bundles of the normal anterior cruciate ligament. *Orthopedics.* 2009;32(9):687–693. https://doi.org/10.3928/01477447-20090728-35.

CHAPTER 3

Anterior Cruciate Ligament Prevention Programs Overview

MATTHEW T. PROVENCHER, MD, CAPT, MC, USNR •
BRENDAN T. HIGGINS, MD, MS • JOHN P. BEGLY, MD • GENEVRA L. STONE, MD •
ANTHONY SANCHEZ, BS • COLIN P. MURPHY, BA

INTRODUCTION

Injuries to the anterior cruciate ligament (ACL) are among the most common knee disorders that require orthopedic surgical intervention. These injuries are particularly prevalent in the young and active population, and ACL injury rates are especially high in female athletes. When compared with males, ACL injury rates are two to eight times higher in females.[1,2] Over the past several decades, female participation in competitive sports has increased dramatically. As this trend continues, the incidence of ACL injuries in female athletes continues to rise.[3] These injuries have significant consequences, both to the athlete and the healthcare system. For the female athlete, an ACL tear entails physical and mental pain, lost athletic opportunities, potential concurrent knee injuries, and long-term morbidity, as well as potential financial implications such as loss of athletic scholarship.[4] In regard to the healthcare system, the lifetime cost of an ACL reconstruction is $38,121/per patient, while the lifetime cost of ACL nonoperative rehabilitation is $88,538/per patient.[3] Given these stakes, much interest and effort has been devoted to the study of ACL injury prevention programs (IPPs).[5]

ACL tears most commonly occur due to a noncontact mechanism. Approximately 70% of all ACL injuries occur in this manner.[6,7] This injury mechanism involves foot strike at or near full extension combined with a forceful valgus and/or tibial rotation moment.[8] Compared with male athletes, female athletes are more likely to be injured from a low-energy noncontact deceleration mechanism rather than from a forceful jump or impact. Injuries sustained in this manner typically occur at lower ground reaction forces.

RISK FACTORS FOR ANTERIOR CRUCIATE LIGAMENT INJURY

Common Nonmodifiable Versus Modifiable Risk Factors

- Nonmodifiable
  - Notch stenosis
  - Ligamentous laxity
  - Tibial plateau slope
  - Hormonal function
  - Neuromuscular maturation
- Modifiable
  - Dynamic knee valgus
  - Quadriceps/hamstring imbalance
  - Decreased core strength
  - Fatigue

Studies have identified multiple risk factors that may place females at a higher risk for ACL tears. Many of these risk factors involve anatomic considerations specific to the female athlete, such as intercondylar notch width, quadriceps/hamstring interaction, ACL size, posterior tibial slope, hyperlaxity, and body mass index.[9,10] Although the discrepancy between ACL injuries in males and females is certainly multifactorial, the landing mechanics of the female athlete contribute significantly to the risk of ACL tears. Compared with males, females land in a more erect position with more knee valgus and increased lower-extremity rotation. Before focusing on the details of prevention strategies and programs, it is essential to understand the pathologic aspects of landing mechanics that place the ACL at risk.

In 2005, Hewett and colleagues[11] performed a cohort analysis of the landing mechanics of over 200 female soccer, basketball, and volleyball players. Mechanics were monitored with three-dimensional (3D) kinematics as well as joint angle and load analysis. Nine athletes in the study sustained ACL tears. These individuals demonstrated significantly different posture and loading during jumping tasks. Additionally, the mean knee abduction angle in the injured athletes was 8 degrees larger than that of controls, and they demonstrated 20% higher ground reaction forces and a stance time that was 16% shorter than controls. Knee abduction moment, which is a measure similar to that of knee valgus, predicted ACL injury in the study with 72% specificity and 78% sensitivity. Increased knee abduction moments

ACL Injuries in Female Athletes. https://doi.org/10.1016/B978-0-323-54839-7.00003-8

correlate to increased valgus during landing, which is a risk factor for noncontact ACL injury. Ligaments on the lateral side of the knee relax, whereas the medial knee tightens, which encourages anterior shift of the lateral tibial plateau and increased ACL strain. Myer et al.[12] demonstrated that athletes with knee abduction moments above 25.3 Nm had a 6.8% risk of ACL tear compared with a 0.4% risk in athletes with values below this threshold. Numata and colleagues[13] examined the biomechanics of 291 high-school female athletes over a 3-year period, and those who sustained an ACL tear demonstrated significantly higher dynamic knee valgus landing moments than the uninjured controls.

Multiple studies have utilized video analysis to investigate the landing mechanics of female athletes. Boden and colleagues demonstrated that subjects with ACL tears first contacted the ground with the hindfoot or flatfoot, whereas healthy controls landed with their forefoot first.[8] Landing with less plantar-flexed ankle angles at the point of contact leads to a shortened stance time and less ability of the calf musculature to absorb ground reaction forces. Additionally, injured subjects landed with significantly higher hip flexion angles. The authors concluded their study by identifying "safe" and "provocative" landing mechanics. Overall, female athletes demonstrated increased knee valgus during landing and cutting, higher knee extension moments, decreased strength in hip abductors, and increased lateral trunk angles. In 3D biomechanical analysis of 171 young female athletes, Leppanen and colleagues[14] illustrated that ACL injuries correlated with lower peak knee flexion angles during landing. Hewett and colleagues[15] performed a similar study and concluded that lateral trunk angle and knee abduction angles were higher in females than in males during ACL injury. High lateral trunk angle causes the center of mass to be displaced to the lateral side of the knee, increasing lateral compartment axial forces and valgus moment during landing.

Similar to Boden, Ireland and colleagues[16] identified "position of safety" and "position of no return" regarding the landing mechanics of female athletes. Safe landing involves normal lordosis of the lumbar spine with the knees flexed. The lower extremity is in overall neutral rotation, as the calf musculature functions to absorb the ground reaction forces of impact. The risk of ACL injury increases when an athlete lands with lumbar flexion, lateral trunk shift, knee extension, and tibial rotation. These factors combine to increase anterior shear and compression force vectors across the knee and result in increased ACL strain. The lower extremity is a kinetic chain that begins in the core musculature and depends upon efficient movement and energy transfer.[17] Weak hip musculature and control contributes to increased valgus landing moments and force vectors across the knee. Zazulak and colleagues[18] examined the biomechanics of 277 collegiate athletes and found that core weakness predicted knee injury; specifically in female athletes, the presence of significant core weakness was 56% specific and 90% sensitive for predicting ACL injury. Similarly, they demonstrated that poor core proprioception also predicted female knee injuries.[19]

Once the biomechanical risk factors for ACL injury are understood, the orthopedic community can focus its attention on the modification of these risk factors in the form of IPPs. All prevention programs must be multifactorial and include strengthening, proprioception, and motion training while emphasizing routine and repetition. It is important to note that a strengthening program alone is not sufficient and does not lead to effective injury prevention.[20]

COMPONENTS OF ANTERIOR CRUCIATE LIGAMENT INJURY PREVENTION PROGRAMS

Many studies have aimed to investigate both the practicality and the success of various ACL IPPs. These programs involve a variety of exercises, several of which are displayed in Table 3.1. Most exercises involve a plyometric component in which muscles exert large forces in short intervals of time with the goal of maximizing power and explosion. The vertical drop jump test is a common component and involves a drop from height followed by an immediate maximal vertical jump (Fig. 3.1). The lateral hop test is also commonly utilized and consists of a one-foot jump onto an elevated surface followed by a jump and a one-leg landing. Each position is held for approximately 3 s, and all movements are performed with a focus on technique and form (Fig. 3.2).

GOALS OF ANTERIOR CRUCIATE LIGAMENT INJURY PREVENTION PROGRAMS

Prevention of Dynamic Knee Valgus/Knee Abduction

Ford et al. studied 81 high-school basketball players (47 female, 34 male) using a drop vertical jump test. Athletes dropped off a box, landed, and immediately performed a maximum vertical jump. The valgus knee moment was analyzed at landing. Female athletes landed with a greater maximum valgus knee angle than male athletes.[23] In a prospective controlled study, Hewett et al.

studied 205 female athletes involved in soccer, basketball, and volleyball. The athletes were evaluated prior to the start of their seasons for neuromuscular control. Of the 205 athletes, 9 subsequently sustained an ACL rupture during their season. In these athletes the knee abduction angle was 8 degrees greater, the knee abduction moment was 2.5 times greater, and the ground reaction force was 20% higher than the uninjured athletes.[11]

Improvement of Quadriceps-Hamstring Balance

Two studies performed at the University of Michigan have helped demonstrate this concept. In the first study,

TABLE 3.1 Typical Exercises Utilized as Part of Anterior Cruciate Ligament Injury Prevention Programs	
ANTERIOR CRUCIATE LIGAMENT INJURY PREVENTION PROGRAM EXERCISES	
Lateral jump	Table lateral crunch
Hop-hold	Table double crunch
BOSU single-knee hold	BOSU single-leg pelvic bridge
Single-leg lateral Airex hop-hold	Back hyperextension with ball reach
Tuck jump	Single-leg 90-degree hop-hold
Walking lunge	Vertical drop jump test

Huston and Wojtys studied 40 female and 60 male athletes and sex-matched controls using isokinetic testing. Dynamic stress testing of muscles demonstrated less anterior tibial translation in athletes (both men and women) compared with nonathletic controls. However, females (athletes and controls) demonstrated more anterior tibial laxity than males. Interestingly, female athletes took longer to generate maximum muscle torque during isokinetic testing and fired their quadriceps first in response to anterior tibial translation, whereas all the other groups, including female controls, fired their hamstrings first.[24] In the second study, which is a cadaver study, Withrow et al. examined 10 knees fixed at 25-degree flexion. The knees were axially loaded with 1700 N to simulate drop landing and cause further knee flexion. They replaced the quadriceps, hamstrings, and gastrocnemius with pretensioned springs. The tension in quadriceps and gastrocnemius was held constant. The tension of the hamstring force was adjustable. They found that increasing the hamstring force decreased the peak relative strain in the ACL by up to 70%.[25] In a study utilizing videographic and electromyographic analyses to analyze knee and hip angular motion patterns, Chappell et al. had 36 recreational athletes (17 men and 19 women) perform vertical stop-jump tasks. Compared with men, women generally exhibited decreased knee flexion, hip flexion, abduction, and external rotation and increased knee internal rotation and quadriceps activation. Interestingly, females exhibited increased

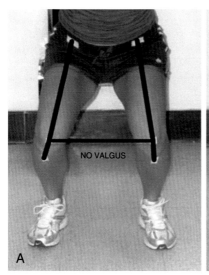 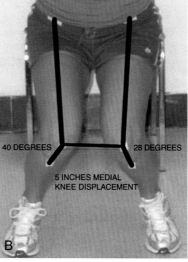

FIG. 3.1 **(A)** Good and **(B)** poor drop jump landing mechanics characterized by dynamic medial collapse of the knees during the landing phase. (Reprinted from Ortiz A, Micheo W. Biomechanical evaluation of the athlete's knee: from basic science to clinical application. *PM R.* 2011;3(4):365–371.)

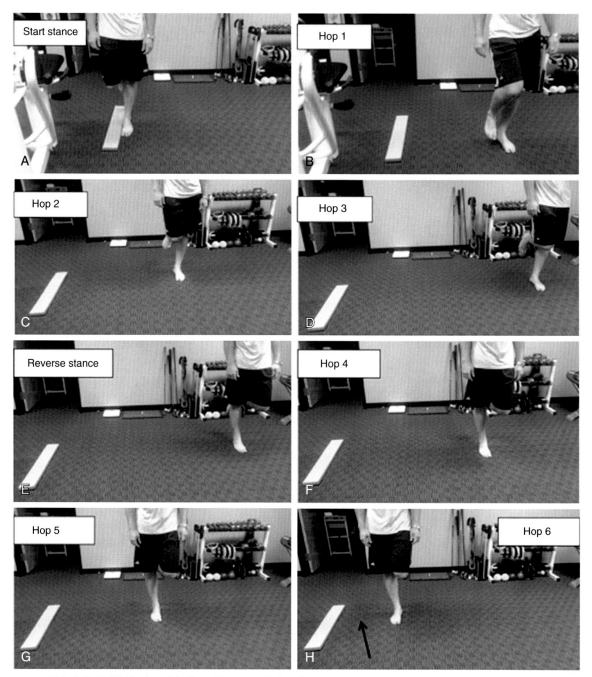

FIG. 3.2 **(A–H)** Version of the lateral hop test. Patient first stands on uninjured leg and takes three successive lateral hops. From this end point the patient then stands on the injured leg and is instructed to take three successive lateral hops back, with the goal of reaching the starting point. *Arrow* depicted in final figure shows failure of the subject to reach the starting point on the injured leg. (Reprinted from Richie DH, Izadi FE. Return to play after an ankle sprain: guidelines for the podiatric physician. *Clin Podiatr Med Surg.* 2015;32(2):195–215.)

hamstring activation before landing but decreased hamstring activation after landing.[26]

Prevention of Core Muscle Weakness/ Lateral Trunk Displacement

Zazulak and colleagues examined the effect of core muscle weakness on ACL injuries. In a study published in 2007, they prospectively followed up 277 collegiate athletes (140 women and 137 men). Athletes were initially placed in an apparatus that stabilized the pelvis. A chest harness with attached cable that applied a force in three different directions was attached and tensioned, forcing the athlete to perform an isometric contraction. The force was then suddenly released and the trunk displacement measured. Over the 3-year follow-up period, 25 of the 277 athletes sustained knee injuries (14 males, 11 females). Six of these were ACL injuries (4 females, 2 males). The 3D trunk displacement was greater in injured athletes, and lateral truck displacement was the strongest predictor of knee injury.[18]

Prevention of Fatigue

Chappell and colleagues examined the effects of fatigue on tibial anterior shear force, varus/valgus moment, and knee flexion angle at peak proximal tibial anterior shear force. They analyzed 20 recreational athletes (10 males, 10 females) performing a jump task with video capture analysis—stop-jump before and after a fatigue-inducing exercise. They found an increased peak proximal tibial anterior shear force, an increased tendency toward valgus, and a decrease in knee flexion angle at peak proximal tibial anterior shear force both in females and in the fatigued state.[27] Additionally, Borotikar et al.[28] quantified the initial contact and peak stance phase 3D lower limb joint kinematics of 25 female National College Athletic Association athletes during anticipated and unanticipated single-leg (left and right) landings, both before and during the accumulation of fatigue. Fatigue was found to cause significant increases in initial contact hip extension and internal rotation, as well as in peak stance knee abduction and internal rotation and ankle supination angles (Fig. 3.3). Fatigue-induced increases

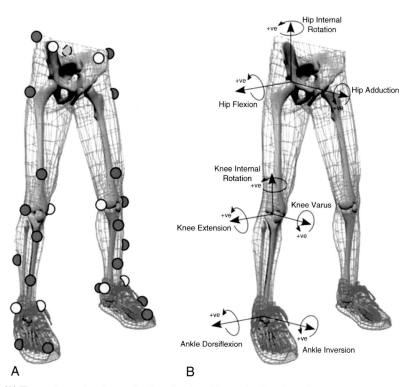

FIG. 3.3 **(A)** Three-dimensional coordinate reflective skin marker locations (28 in total; 12.7 mm diameter) used to quantify lower limb joint landing rotations. **(B)** The hip, knee, and ankle joints were each assigned three rotational directions of force. (Reprinted from Borotikar BS, Newcomer R, Koppes R, McLean SG. Combined effects of fatigue and decision making on female lower limb landing postures: central and peripheral contributions to ACL injury risk. *Clin Biomech (Bristol, Avon)*. 2008;23(1):81–92.)

in initial contact hip rotations and peak knee abduction angle were also significantly more pronounced during unanticipated than during anticipated landings.

PUBLISHED PREVENTION PROGRAMS AND EVIDENCE OF EFFICACY

Biomechanical Outcomes

One of the first ACL IPPs was performed at the University of Cincinnati and examined the effects of plyometric training on landing forces, knee abduction, and hamstring power. This was a before-after study in which 11 female high-school volleyball players performed a drop landing task before and after a 6-week plyometric training program. On average, peak landing force decreased 22%, knee abduction decreased 50%, and hamstring muscle power increased 44% on the dominant side and 21% on the nondominant side. Additionally, peak vertical jump height increased 10%, showing that these programs not only can decrease injury risk but also may improve performance.[29]

The same group then compared plyometric training with dynamic stabilization and balance training. A total of 18 high-school female athletes underwent a 7-week training program. Of them, 8 athletes focused on plyometric exercises and 10 on dynamic stabilization and balance exercises. Lower-extremity kinematics were analyzed using 3D video motion analysis during a drop vertical jump. Those athletes who underwent plyometric training had a greater knee flexion angle upon landing. However, the athletes who underwent dynamic stabilization and resistance training displayed a greater effect in regard to decreased hip adduction, knee abduction, and ankle eversion. Perhaps, this study gives evidence to the need for both balance training to improve coronal plane mechanics and plyometric training to improve sagittal plane mechanics.[30] In a cluster-randomized study performed at the United States Military Academy, DiStefano et al.[31] found that although an IPP is likely beneficial, a maintenance program is necessary for sustained benefit.

Clinical Outcomes

Hewett and colleagues[32] were the first to demonstrate that targeted neuromuscular training (TNMT) programs can reduce the risk of ACL tears. The authors performed a prospective cohort study on high-school female athletes. The athletes participated in a TNMT IPP performed over a 6-week period. The program consisted of three 60- to 90-min sessions per week. Noncontact ACL tear risk was found to be significantly lower in the trained athletes. Athletes who completed

the program demonstrated a 72% reduction when compared with untrained controls. None of the athletes who completed the program sustained an ACL tear. The authors concluded that effective ACL IPPs should ideally include technique training in the setting of plyometric exercises and be performed more than once a week for at least 6 weeks.

Myklebust et al.[33] also examined the efficacy of ACL prevention programs in a prospective cohort study performed over 3 years. The study population consisted of over 850 Norwegian female handball players, who were followed up over three seasons. An ACL IPP was implemented in seasons two and three of the study. In the first season, 29 ACL injuries occurred, prior to intervention, which served as the study control. In seasons two and three, 23 and 17 ACL injuries occurred, respectively. Overall, there was a significant reduction in noncontact ACL tears following implementation of the IPP, particularly in elite division athletes. When normalized for exposure, the authors demonstrated a 36% lower risk of ACL tears in athletes who then completed training intervention.

Several studies have contributed to the development of the FIFA 11+ program, which is an ACL IPP with documented success when used in soccer players.[34,35] The program consists of running, strengthening, plyometric, and balance exercises. Typically, it is performed during a team warm-up routine and was designed to be supervised by the team coach. There are three performance levels for each exercise, all of which emphasize correct lower extremity and trunk alignment. Other than cones, no additional equipment is necessary to complete the exercises. In comparison, many of the TNMT programs differ in several respects from the FIFA 11+ program. TNMT programs typically focus less on running and more on plyometric exercises and are supervised by an athletic trainer.[36] Additionally, often there are more levels of performance to allow for further advancement and refinement of technique, as well as equipment that provides an unstable support during exercises, creating a more challenging training environment and activating additional supporting accessory musculature and soft tissue stabilizers.

Mandelbaum and colleagues[37] examined the effectiveness of TNMT and proprioceptive training programs in the prevention of ACL injuries in female soccer players. Over 1000 players and matched controls were included in the study, and athletes were followed up over two seasons. Training interventions significantly decreased the incidence of ACL tears per 1000 player exposures. Overall, there were only six ACL tears in the trained group, compared with 67 tears in the untrained controls. Petersen et al.[38] performed a similar prospective study on prevention programs in female German handball athletes. A total of 10 teams completed the ACL prevention training program and were compared with 10 control teams. The program consisted of exercises performed on a balance board and bounce mat, as well as explosive jumps. ACL injury risk was 80% lower in the trained group.

Hewett and colleagues[36] investigated the effectiveness of TNMT in relation to the individual neuromuscular risk profile of female athletes. The specific TNMT program utilized in the study included a drop vertical jump, single-leg drop, and single-leg cross jump exercises. There was no running component and the program was supervised by an athletic trainer. Athletes' performance in jumping, cutting, and pivoting tasks was assessed before and after TMNT. Participation in the TNMT program significantly improved both hip control and peak trunk flexion angles. These results were confirmed by Pollard and colleagues,[39] who reported improved knee landing mechanics, trunk flexion angles, and lower-extremity energy absorption in female soccer players who completed a 12-week TNMT program. Hewett demonstrated that high-risk athletes improved more than low-risk athletes, suggesting that individuals with high baseline risk profiles may benefit the most from participating in an ACL IPP.

Meta-Analyses and Systematic Reviews

In a 2010 meta-analysis of seven published studies, Yoo et al. found an odds ratio of 0.4 [95% confidence interval (CI), 0.27–0.60] in favor of prevention programs. Subgroup analyses identified age <18 years, soccer, a combined preseason and in-season program, and plyometric and strengthening exercises over balance training as factors that favored prevention.[40] In a 2012 meta-analysis, Sadoghi et al. found a 0.38 (95% CI, 0.2–0.72) pooled risk ratio in favor of prevention programs. They showed a 52% risk reduction among male athletes and an 85% risk reduction among female athletes. They did not find any evidence to support any one specific intervention program.[41] Lopes et al.[42] conducted a systematic review examining the effects of IPPs on the biomechanics of landing tasks. A total of 28 studies including 466 subjects were analyzed, and IPPs were found to significantly decrease peak knee abduction moments. The authors concluded that prevention programs allow athletes to improve lower-extremity control and more effectively accommodate ligament imbalances during landing tasks, which in turn decreases potential compromising strain on the ACL.

COMPLIANCE/SUPERVISION

Pfile et al. examined the need for supervision while performing an ACL IPP. They looked at the number needed to treat (NNT) for peer-led, coach-led, or coach and healthcare provider (team-led) programs. They found that coach-led (NNT = 120) and team-led (NNT = 133) programs were superior to peer-led programs. They felt that a well-trained coach can adequately supervise an IPP.[43] In a study by Thein-Nissenbaum et al. examining the barriers to compliance in an 8-week home-based ACL IPP in high-school female athletes, only 27 of 66 athletes who were given the program responded to the questionnaire. Of the 27 who did respond, only 3 (11%) performed the exercises for the recommended 3 days per week.[44]

LINK BETWEEN INJURY PREVENTION AND PERFORMANCE

Myer et al. showed that in addition to improvements in the valgus torque of the knee, completing an ACL IPP had a significant increase in maximum squat strength and single-leg hop distance and improvement in sprint times. For maximum athlete and coach buy-in, the ACL IPP should link injury prevention with increased performance.[45]

SHOULD WE BE SCREENING?

Myer et al. were the first to examine the possibility of screening female athletes and creating high-risk and low-risk groups. Groups were identified through motion analysis of a drop vertical jump and calculation of knee abduction moment. There was a significant decrease in knee abduction moment in the "high-risk" group but no decrease in the "low-risk" group following a training program.[46] In 2009, DiStefano et al. performed a similar study. They used the Landing Error Scoring System as a screening tool to evaluate 173 middle- and high-school-aged soccer players. They found that the athletes with the greatest amount of movement errors experienced the most improvement after a neuromuscular program.[47] The American Academy of Orthopedic Surgeons (AAOS) has created a web-based tool that will provide guidance on the utility of IPPs for athletes based on sex, pubertal status, level of activity, what sports they participate in, and athlete risk as per the screening evaluation.[48]

COST-EFFECTIVENESS

Swart et al. examined the cost-effectiveness of ACL screening and IPPs. They concluded, "Given its low cost and ease of implementation, neuromuscular training of all young athletes represents a cost-effective strategy for reducing costs and morbidity from ACL injuries. While continued innovations on inexpensive and accurate screening methods to identify high-risk athletes remain of interest, improving existing training protocols and implementing neuromuscular training into routine training for all young athletes is warranted." Additionally, the study offers good evidence that screening programs are not as cost-effective as universal training programs.[49]

CONCLUSION

Overall, the evidence provided by these studies and others has led to a moderate-strength-evidence recommendation to support the use of ACL IPPs according to the AAOS Evidence-Based Clinical Guidelines for ACL injuries.[50] The length of intervention is integral to the success of any ACL IPP. Padua and colleagues[51] demonstrated this very important finding in their study, in which they compared the retention of biomechanical improvements in two groups who completed an IPP. One group performed the program for 3 months, whereas the second group performed the program for 9 months. Both groups demonstrated improved performance, but only the extended duration group maintained these gains 3 months after stopping the program. The study illustrated that the benefits gained from participation in an ACL IPP fade with discontinuation of the program.

As mentioned previously, the baseline risk profile of a female athlete influences an athlete's response to TNMT intervention. ACL IPPs are most beneficial in younger individuals, higher-risk athletes, and athletes who perform at an elite level.[52] Programs that identify base line risk factors of participants have the best chance of achieving the desired effectiveness in regard to injury prevention.

As the study of ACL injury prevention continues to progress, advancements in real-time data collection and analysis will likely be useful components to the future of TNMT programs. Wearable technology has already become more common in our society, and it represents a potentially valuable resource in the continued development of IPPs. Decker and colleagues[53] have examined the use of wearable neuromuscular devices in ACL IPPs. The device was used to measure posture and ground reaction forces during athletic activities in female soccer players. Players demonstrated biomechanical improvements after participation in the prevention program with the device, and the NNT to prevent one ACL injury was 92. Future studies aimed at

optimizing the practicality and usefulness of wearable technology will be valuable to the continued improvement of ACL IPPs.

An important question surrounding ACL IPPs is how to best implement these interventions in a practical and effective manner. In today's world, young athletes are surrounded by stressors, from the classroom to their home to their social circle. With pressures on their time from a multitude of directions, it can be difficult to find time to perform a dedicated program several times a week. Integration of the program into a team's standard practice routine, such as during a warm-up with all athletes included, may be a more practical option for program implementation rather than performing the regimen at a separate time. Currently, there are no widely accepted recommendations regarding the details of practical implementation, and together athletes, coaches, parents, and medical personnel should work to establish a plan that optimizes the ability to complete the IPP both efficiently and effectively.

ACL IPPs are effective in decreasing the incidence of ACL tears among female athletes, particularly in young elite-level athletes with baseline risk factors for ACL injury. The most effective programs incorporate a combination of training exercises and standardized schedule (Table 3.2). Programs should ideally include plyometric, proprioceptive, and technique training

TABLE 3.2
Components of a Valuable Anterior Cruciate Ligament Injury Prevention Program and Populations Where They are Most Effective

ACL injury prevention programs most effective in	Younger athletes
	Higher-risk athletes
	Elite performance athletes
Components of a valuable ACL injury prevention program	Dynamic strengthening of the lower-extremity kinetic chain
	Plyometric and proprioceptive training
	Technique training
	Multiple sessions per week 10 min each for 3 sessions for a week minimum
	Preseason implementation
	Continued participation in season
	Longer duration of intervention
	Identification of at-risk athletes

ACL, anterior cruciate ligament.

aimed at dynamic strengthening of the lower-extremity kinetic chain. Additionally, programs should be performed multiple times a week. The minimum recommendation is at least 10 min per session three times per week, but longer sessions are more beneficial. Programs should be implemented before the competitive season begins, and athletes with high baseline risk profiles should be identified at this time. Finally, programs should be continued throughout the season and the intervention should be continued for as long as possible because the biomechanical benefits of ACL prevention programs fade with discontinuation of program participation.

SUMMARY

- Literature supports the use of ACL IPPs
- Should incorporate plyometric, balance, resistance, and neuromuscular modalities to prevent
  - dynamic knee valgus
  - quadriceps dominance
  - leg dominance
  - core/trunk muscle weakness
  - fatigue
- Should be supervised
- Should incorporate video feedback when possible
- Should be year-round—both preseason and in season
- Should be aligned with improved performance

REFERENCES

1. Snaebjornsson T, Hamrin Senorski E, Sundemo D, et al. Adolescents and female patients are at increased risk for contralateral anterior cruciate ligament reconstruction: a cohort study from the Swedish National Knee Ligament Register based on 17,682 patients. *Knee Surg Sports Traumatol Arthrosc.* 2017;25(12):3938–3944.
2. Toth AP, Cordasco FA. Anterior cruciate ligament injuries in the female athlete. *J Gend Specif Med.* 2001;4(4):25–34.
3. Mather 3rd RC, Koenig L, Kocher MS, et al. Societal and economic impact of anterior cruciate ligament tears. *J Bone Joint Surg Am.* 2013;95(19):1751–1759.
4. Giugliano DN, Solomon JL. ACL tears in female athletes. *Phys Med Rehabil Clin N Am.* 2007;18(3):417–438, viii.
5. Hewett TE, Myer GD, Ford KR. Anterior cruciate ligament injuries in female athletes: part 1, mechanisms and risk factors. *Am J Sports Med.* 2006;34(2):299–311.
6. Boden BP, Dean GS, Feagin Jr JA, Garrett Jr WE. Mechanisms of anterior cruciate ligament injury. *Orthopedics.* 2000;23(6):573–578.
7. McNair PJ, Marshall RN, Matheson JA. Important features associated with acute anterior cruciate ligament injury. *N Z Med J.* 1990;103(901):537–539.
8. Boden BP, Torg JS, Knowles SB, Hewett TE. Video analysis of anterior cruciate ligament injury: abnormalities in hip and ankle kinematics. *Am J Sports Med.* 2009;37(2):252–259.
9. Boden BP, Sheehan FT, Torg JS, Hewett TE. Noncontact anterior cruciate ligament injuries: mechanisms and risk factors. *J Am Acad Orthop Surg.* 2010;18(9):520–527.
10. Renstrom P, Ljungqvist A, Arendt E, et al. Non-contact ACL injuries in female athletes: an International Olympic Committee current concepts statement. *Br J Sports Med.* 2008;42(6):394–412.
11. Hewett TE, Myer GD, Ford KR, et al. Biomechanical measures of neuromuscular control and valgus loading of the knee predict anterior cruciate ligament injury risk in female athletes: a prospective study. *Am J Sports Med.* 2005;33(4):492–501.
12. Myer GD, Ford KR, Di Stasi SL, Foss KD, Micheli LJ, Hewett TE. High knee abduction moments are common risk factors for patellofemoral pain (PFP) and anterior cruciate ligament (ACL) injury in girls: is PFP itself a predictor for subsequent ACL injury? *Br J Sports Med.* 2015;49(2):118–122.
13. Numata H, Nakase J, Kitaoka K, et al. Two-dimensional motion analysis of dynamic knee valgus identifies female high school athletes at risk of non-contact anterior cruciate ligament injury. *Knee Surg Sports Traumatol Arthrosc.* 2018;26(2):442–447.
14. Leppanen M, Pasanen K, Kujala UM, et al. Stiff landings are associated with increased ACL injury risk in young female basketball and floorball players. *Am J Sports Med.* 2017;45(2):386–393.
15. Hewett TE, Torg JS, Boden BP. Video analysis of trunk and knee motion during non-contact anterior cruciate ligament injury in female athletes: lateral trunk and knee abduction motion are combined components of the injury mechanism. *Br J Sports Med.* 2009;43(6):417–422.
16. Ireland ML, Ballantyne BT, Little K, McClay IS. A radiographic analysis of the relationship between the size and shape of the intercondylar notch and anterior cruciate ligament injury. *Knee Surg Sports Traumatol Arthrosc.* 2001;9(4):200–205.
17. Ford KR, Myer GD, Hewett TE. Longitudinal effects of maturation on lower extremity joint stiffness in adolescent athletes. *Am J Sports Med.* 2010;38(9):1829–1837.
18. Zazulak BT, Hewett TE, Reeves NP, Goldberg B, Cholewicki J. Deficits in neuromuscular control of the trunk predict knee injury risk: a prospective biomechanical-epidemiologic study. *Am J Sports Med.* 2007;35(7):1123–1130.
19. Zazulak BT, Hewett TE, Reeves NP, Goldberg B, Cholewicki J. The effects of core proprioception on knee injury: a prospective biomechanical-epidemiological study. *Am J Sports Med.* 2007;35(3):368–373.
20. Herman DC, Weinhold PS, Guskiewicz KM, Garrett WE, Yu B, Padua DA. The effects of strength training on the lower extremity biomechanics of female recreational athletes during a stop-jump task. *Am J Sports Med.* 2008;36(4):733–740.

21. Ortiz A, Micheo W. Biomechanical evaluation of the athlete's knee: from basic science to clinical application. *PM R*. 2011;3(4):365–371.

22. Richie DH, Izadi FE. Return to play after an ankle sprain: guidelines for the podiatric physician. *Clin Podiatr Med Surg*. 2015;32(2):195–215.

23. Ford KR, Myer GD, Hewett TE. Valgus knee motion during landing in high school female and male basketball players. *Med Sci Sports Exerc*. 2003;35(10):1745–1750.

24. Huston LJ, Wojtys EM. Neuromuscular performance characteristics in elite female athletes. *Am J Sports Med*. 1996;24(4):427–436.

25. Withrow TJ, Huston LJ, Wojtys EM, Ashton-Miller JA. Effect of varying hamstring tension on anterior cruciate ligament strain during in vitro impulsive knee flexion and compression loading. *J Bone Joint Surg Am*. 2008;90(4):815–823.

26. Chappell JD, Creighton RA, Giuliani C, Yu B, Garrett WE. Kinematics and electromyography of landing preparation in vertical stop-jump: risks for noncontact anterior cruciate ligament injury. *Am J Sports Med*. 2007;35(2):235–241.

27. Chappell JD, Herman DC, Knight BS, Kirkendall DT, Garrett WE, Yu B. Effect of fatigue on knee kinetics and kinematics in stop-jump tasks. *Am J Sports Med*. 2005;33(7):1022–1029.

28. Borotikar BS, Newcomer R, Koppes R, McLean SG. Combined effects of fatigue and decision making on female lower limb landing postures: central and peripheral contributions to ACL injury risk. *Clin Biomech (Bristol Avon)*. 2008;23(1):81–92.

29. Hewett TE, Stroupe AL, Nance TA, Noyes FR. Plyometric training in female athletes. Decreased impact forces and increased hamstring torques. *Am J Sports Med*. 1996;24(6):765–773.

30. Myer GD, Ford KR, McLean SG, Hewett TE. The effects of plyometric versus dynamic stabilization and balance training on lower extremity biomechanics. *Am J Sports Med*. 2006;34(3):445–455.

31. DiStefano LJ, Marshall SW, Padua DA, et al. The effects of an injury prevention program on landing biomechanics over time. *Am J Sports Med*. 2016;44(3):767–776.

32. Hewett TE, Lindenfeld TN, Riccobene JV, Noyes FR. The effect of neuromuscular training on the incidence of knee injury in female athletes. A prospective study. *Am J Sports Med*. 1999;27(6):699–706.

33. Myklebust G, Engebretsen L, Braekken IH, Skjolberg A, Olsen OE, Bahr R. Prevention of anterior cruciate ligament injuries in female team handball players: a prospective intervention study over three seasons. *Clin J Sport Med*. 2003;13(2):71–78.

34. Junge A, Lamprecht M, Stamm H, et al. Countrywide campaign to prevent soccer injuries in Swiss amateur players. *Am J Sports Med*. 2011;39(1):57–63.

35. Myklebust G, Skjolberg A, Bahr R. ACL injury incidence in female handball 10 years after the Norwegian ACL prevention study: important lessons learned. *Br J Sports Med*. 2013;47(8):476–479.

36. Hewett TE, Ford KR, Xu YY, Khoury J, Myer GD. Effectiveness of neuromuscular training based on the neuromuscular risk profile. *Am J Sports Med*. 2017;45(9):2142–2147.

37. Mandelbaum BR, Silvers HJ, Watanabe DS, et al. Effectiveness of a neuromuscular and proprioceptive training program in preventing anterior cruciate ligament injuries in female athletes: 2-year follow-up. *Am J Sports Med*. 2005;33(7):1003–1010.

38. Petersen W, Braun C, Bock W, et al. A controlled prospective case control study of a prevention training program in female team handball players: the German experience. *Arch Orthop Trauma Surg*. 2005;125(9):614–621.

39. Pollard CD, Sigward SM, Powers CM. ACL injury prevention training results in modification of hip and knee mechanics during a drop-landing task. *Orthop J Sports Med*. 2017;5.

40. Yoo JH, Lim BO, Ha M, et al. A meta-analysis of the effect of neuromuscular training on the prevention of the anterior cruciate ligament injury in female athletes. *Knee Surg Sports Traumatol Arthrosc*. 2010;18(6):824–830.

41. Sadoghi P, von Keudell A, Vavken P. Effectiveness of anterior cruciate ligament injury prevention training programs. *J Bone Joint Surg Am*. 2012;94(9):769–776.

42. Lopes TJA, Simic M, Myer GD, Ford KR, Hewett TE, Pappas E. The effects of injury prevention programs on the biomechanics of landing tasks: a systematic review with meta-analysis. *Am J Sports Med*. 2017:363546517716930.

43. Pfile KR, Curioz B. Coach-led prevention programs are effective in reducing anterior cruciate ligament injury risk in female athletes: a number-needed-to-treat analysis. *Scand J Med Sci Sports*. 2017;27(12):1950–1958.

44. Thein-Nissenbaum J, Brooks MA. Barriers to compliance in a home-based anterior cruciate ligament injury prevention program in female high school athletes. *WMJ*. 2016;115(1):37–42.

45. Myer GD, Ford KR, Palumbo JP, Hewett TE. Neuromuscular training improves performance and lower-extremity biomechanics in female athletes. *J Strength Cond Res*. 2005;19(1):51–60.

46. Myer GD, Ford KR, Brent JL, Hewett TE. Differential neuromuscular training effects on ACL injury risk factors in "high-risk" versus "low-risk" athletes. *BMC Musculoskelet Disord*. 2007;8:39.

47. DiStefano LJ, Padua DA, DiStefano MJ, Marshall SW. Influence of age, sex, technique, and exercise program on movement patterns after an anterior cruciate ligament injury prevention program in youth soccer players. *Am J Sports Med*. 2009;37(3):495–505.

48. Sanders JO, Brown GA, Murray J, Pezold R, Sevarino K. Anterior cruciate ligament injury prevention programs. *J Am Acad Orthop Surg*. 2017;25(4):e79–e82.

49. Swart E, Redler L, Fabricant PD, Mandelbaum BR, Ahmad CS, Wang YC. Prevention and screening programs for anterior cruciate ligament injuries in young athletes: a cost-effectiveness analysis. *J Bone Joint Surg Am*. 2014;96(9):705–711.

50. Carey JL, Shea KG. AAOS clinical practice guideline: management of anterior cruciate ligament injuries: evidence-based guideline. *J Am Acad Orthop Surg.* 2015;23(5):e6–e8.
51. Padua DA, DiStefano LJ, Marshall SW, Beutler AI, de la Motte SJ, DiStefano MJ. Retention of movement pattern changes after a lower extremity injury prevention program is affected by program duration. *Am J Sports Med.* 2012;40(2):300–306.
52. Myer GD, Sugimoto D, Thomas S, Hewett TE. The influence of age on the effectiveness of neuromuscular training to reduce anterior cruciate ligament injury in female athletes: a meta-analysis. *Am J Sports Med.* 2013;41(1):203–215.
53. Decker MJ, Shaw M, Maddan C, Campbell J, Davidson B. A wearable neuromuscular device reduces ACL injury risk in female soccer athletes. *Orthop J Sports Med.* 2016;4.

CHAPTER 4

Anterior Cruciate Ligament Anatomy

MARCIO ALBERS, MD • MONIQUE C. CHAMBERS, MD, MSL •
ANDREW J. SHEEAN, MD • FREDDIE H. FU, MD, DSC (HON), DPS (HON)

INTRODUCTION

The anterior cruciate ligament (ACL) is of critical importance to the normal function of the knee joint. It has a fundamental role in providing knee stability, particularly during intense activities that require cutting and pivoting movements. Young active individuals, particularly young female athletes, are at increased risk of ACL tears.[1-4] In the United States, more than 130,000 ACL reconstructions (ACLRs) are performed annually with the ultimate goal of restoring knee stability and avoiding associated injuries to the menisci and articular cartilage, which can lead to the development of early osteoarthritis.[5-8]

Over the past decades, a myriad of approaches have been described in the treatment of ACL injuries, ranging from nonanatomic surgeries, such as capsular reefing and extra-articular tenodesis, to the most modern of approaches, such as individualized anatomic ACLR.[9-12] A deeper understanding of the ACL native anatomy is paramount for orthopedic surgeons to be able to deal with multiple aspects involved in determining the best treatment option for each patient. This chapter provides an overview of the key aspects of the ACL anatomy, with special emphasis on the unique characteristics of the female knee.

EMBRYOLOGY

ACL can be identified in the fetus as early as 8 weeks of gestational age.[13-16] Histologic analysis has identified the presence of a distinct ligamentous structure in the intercondylar area of the fetal knee. At 11 weeks of gestational age, microscopic dissection of the fetal ACL, its synovial coverage, and the menisci is possible. After 16 weeks of gestational age, two functional bundles of the ACL, namely, the anteromedial (AM) and the posterolateral (PL) bundles, can be observed (Fig. 4.1).[17] While the fetal ACL bears a strong resemblance to that of adults, there is a greater degree of bundle parallelism in the fetal ACL than that in the adult ACL.[18] This observation may be attributable to the fact that the fetal ACL has not yet been exposed to functional loads

during in utero development. Histologically, it is possible to identify the rich collagen fiber bundles separated by a septum that is rich in neurovascular supply and viable stem cells.[19,20]

GROSS ANATOMY

The ACL is a complex shaped structure that connects the medial wall of the lateral femoral condyle to the central area of the tibial plateau. The ACL double bundle anatomy can be better appreciated from an anterior point of view with the knee flexed to at least 90 degrees (Fig. 4.2). In this position the PL bundle is positioned more posterior and lateral on the tibial insertion site and more anterior on the femoral insertion site, whereas the AM bundle is positioned more anterior and medial on the tibial side and more posterior on the femoral side (Fig. 4.3).[10,21-24]

The ACL tibial insertion site is oval, occupying a broad area between the tibial spines. The length of the ACL tibial insertion varies considerably in the population, averaging 17 ± 2 mm. The AM bundle length and width were on average 9.1 ± 1.2 mm and 9.2 ± 1.1 mm, while the PL bundle measured on average 7.4 ± 1.0 mm and 7.0 ± 1 mm, respectively. Although a positive correlation between the ACL insertion site length and the self-reported height and weight was found, the coefficients of determination were low.[25] The anterior horn of the lateral meniscus has a close relationship with the PL bundle tibial insertion, where their fibers overlap (Fig. 4.4).[26] The width of the ACL tibial insertion is predicated upon the bony morphology of the femoral intercondylar notch, as narrow intercondylar notches have been observed to correlate with ACLs of smaller diameters (Figs. 4.5 and Fig. 4.6).[27,28] Guenther et al. compared the preoperative imaging and intraoperative measurements of the tibial insertion site. The tibial footprint area was on average 123.8 ± 21.5 mm², ranging from 75 to 175 mm².[29]

The ACL isthmus has also been studied extensively. Fujimaki et al. used a robotic system and laser scan to quantify the ACL morphology, correlating the size of the tibial insertion site with the isthmus and femoral

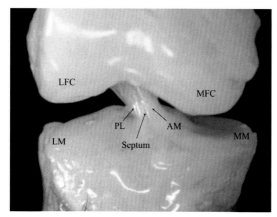

FIG. 4.1 The knee of a fetus at 16 weeks' gestation showing the anterior cruciate ligament bundle anatomy. *AM*, anteromedial; *LFC*, lateral femoral condyle; *LM*, lateral meniscus; *MFC*, medial femoral condyle; *MM*, medial meniscus; *PL*, posterolateral.

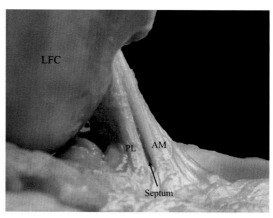

FIG. 4.2 The anterior cruciate ligament anteromedial (AM) and posterolateral (PL) bundles separated by the septum. *LFC*, lateral femoral condyle.

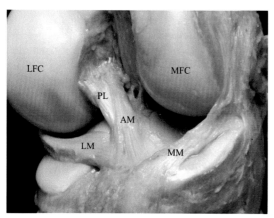

FIG. 4.3 Macroscopic anatomy of the anterior cruciate ligament. *AM*, anteromedial; *LFC*, lateral femoral condyle; *LM*, lateral meniscus; *MFC*, medial femoral condyle; *MM*, medial meniscus; *PL*, posterolateral.

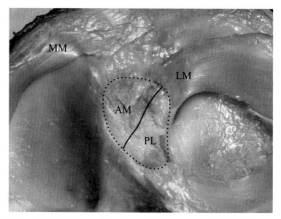

FIG. 4.4 Tibial insertion site. *AM*, anteromedial; *LM*, lateral meniscus; *MM*, medial meniscus; *PL*, posterolateral.

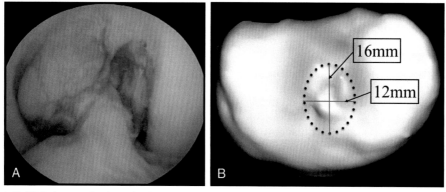

FIG. 4.5 **(A)** Arthroscopic view of a C-shaped femoral intercondylar notch. **(B)** The intraoperative tibial insertion site measurements.

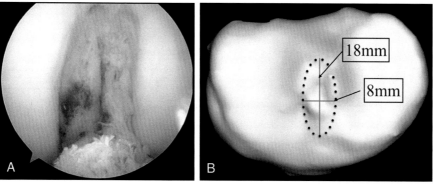

FIG. 4.6 **(A)** Arthroscopic view of an A-shaped femoral intercondylar notch. **(B)** The intraoperative tibial insertion site measurements.

insertion site. The ACL midportion cross-sectional area measured $39.9 \pm 13.7 \, mm^2$ in the unloaded state, while the tibial and femoral insertion sites measured $90.1 \pm 27.4 \, mm^2$ and $118.4 \pm 36.7 \, mm^2$, respectively.[30] Furthermore, the same study provided evidence to suggest that the shape of the isthmus varies dynamically according to the magnitude and direction of the applied loads.

The osseous anatomy of the femoral insertion corroborates the two-bundle concept and is of critical importance to anatomic reconstruction. The lateral intercondylar ridge, which runs from proximal to distal and defines the anterior limits of the ACL femoral insertion site, has been identified in both fetal and adult specimens.[31] The authors described the lateral bifurcate ridge as the bony prominence that separates the insertions of the PL and AM bundles and noted a change in slope of 27 degrees between the insertion of each bundle. The area of the PL and AM bundles was measured to be 120 and $77 \, mm^2$, respectively (Fig. 4.7).[31] Sasaki et al. showed that the fanning-like posterior fibers of the femoral insertion site of the ACL are composed primarily of indirect fibers.[32] Iwahashi et al.[33] studied the femoral insertion site with computerized tomography and histologic analysis, observing that the area in proximity to the lateral intercondylar ridge contains the majority of direct fibers of the ACL. However, specimens used in this study were preserved in formalin and the mean age of the specimens was 70 and 77 years, respectively, which may limit the external validity of these conclusions.[34]

RADIOLOGIC ANATOMY

ACL anatomy is best studied by magnetic resonance imaging (MRI), and a multidimensional understanding of ACL morphology can be enriched by the use

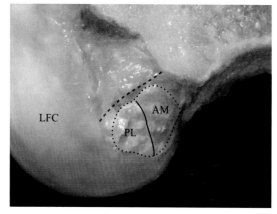

FIG. 4.7 Femoral insertion site. The lateral intercondylar ridge limits the anterior portion of the anterior cruciate ligament (*traced line*). The lateral bifurcate ridge separates the posterolateral (PL) and anteromedial (AM) bundles' footprint (*solid line*). *LFC*, lateral femoral condyle.

of multiple MRI sequences. From these sequences, measurements can be taken and nuances pertaining to patients' unique anatomy can be appreciated.[35–37] The sagittal oblique sequence aligned parallel with the ACL allows for reliable evaluation of the two functional bundles AM and PL, which can be of particular importance in the setting of single-bundle tear patterns (Fig. 4.8).[36] The coronal oblique sequence is useful for visualization of the length of the ACL, as well as both the tibial and femoral insertion sites (Fig. 4.9).[35,37–39]

FEMALE ANTERIOR CRUCIATE LIGAMENT ANATOMY

Given the fact that young active women appear to be at increased risk of ACL tear when compared with

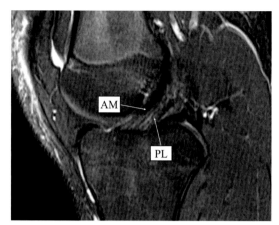

FIG. 4.8 Sagittal T2 magnetic resonance image of the anterior cruciate ligament. *AM*, anteromedial; *PL*, posterolateral.

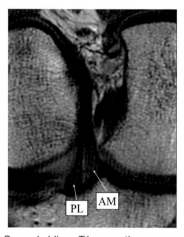

FIG. 4.9 Coronal oblique T1 magnetic resonance image of the anterior cruciate ligament. *AM*, anteromedial; *PL*, posterolateral.

matched cohorts of men, a number of authors have sought to identify particularities of the female ACL that may explain these observed discrepancies.[2–4,28,40–45] Using MRI measurements and correcting for subjects' weight, Anderson et al. showed that the female ACL cross-sectional area measured by MRI averaged to 36.1 mm², whereas the male control group ACL cross-sectional area measured on average 48.9 mm². When the data was controlled for total body weight, significant differences were still present; however, when the data was normalized by lean mass, no significant differences were appreciated.[46]

The smaller size of the female ACL may have implications on the mechanical tissue properties that

contribute to increased rates of injury.[28,47–49] Chandrashekar et al. showed that the mechanical properties of ACL in women are intrinsically lower than those in men. The modulus of elasticity was 22.49% lower, the strain at failure was 8.3% lower, and the stress at failure was 14.3% lower.[50]

Variability in the intercondylar notch dimensions may also contribute to increased ACL injury rates among women. Impingement of the ACL against the intercondylar notch may lead to attritional changes that degrade structural properties and predispose the tissue to failure. Anthropomorphic data has elucidated several important differences in intercondylar notch dimension as a function of gender. Anderson et al. observed that intercondylar notch width increases as a function of height in men, but not in women. Thus taller women may have comparatively narrower intercondylar notches and proportionally smaller ACL.[46] It has also been observed that patients who sustained bilateral ACL tears had narrower notches than those who had unilateral injury.[52] However, this notion is somewhat controversial as van Eck et al. [51] observed no difference in the notch volume measured by MRI between the ACL injury cohort and matched controls.

CONCLUSION

The understanding of the ACL complex anatomy is key for surgeons who would like to follow the modern principles of anatomic ACLR to treat their patients. It is also important in determining the anatomic risk factors that may be identifiable early enough to allow for preventive strategies to be employed, with the goal of providing optimum care for our patients.

REFERENCES

1. Burnham JM, Wright V. Update on anterior cruciate ligament rupture and care in the female athlete. *Clin Sports Med.* 2017;36(4):703–715.
2. Cheung EC, Boguszewski DV, Joshi NB, Wang D, McAllister DR. Anatomic factors that may predispose female athletes to anterior cruciate ligament injury. *Curr Sports Med Rep.* 2015;14(5):368–372.
3. Sugimoto D, Myer GD, Micheli LJ, Hewett TE. ABCs of evidence-based anterior cruciate ligament injury prevention strategies in female athletes. *Curr Phys Med Rehabil Rep.* 2015;3(1):43–49.
4. Uhorchak JM, Scoville CR, Williams GN, Arciero RA, St Pierre P, Taylor DC. Risk factors associated with noncontact injury of the anterior cruciate ligament: a prospective four-year evaluation of 859 West Point cadets. *Am J Sports Med.* 2003;31(6):831–842.

5. Mall NA, Chalmers PN, Moric M, et al. Incidence and trends of anterior cruciate ligament reconstruction in the United States. *Am J Sports Med.* 2014;42(10):2363–2370.
6. van Eck CF, Widhalm H, Murawski C, Fu FH. Individualized anatomic anterior cruciate ligament reconstruction. *Phys Sportsmed.* 2015;43(1):87–92.
7. Moksnes H, Engebretsen L, Risberg MA. Prevalence and incidence of new meniscus and cartilage injuries after a nonoperative treatment algorithm for ACL tears in skeletally immature children: a prospective MRI study. *Am J Sports Med.* 2013;41(8):1771–1779.
8. Sanders TL, Pareek A, Kremers HM, et al. Long-term follow-up of isolated ACL tears treated without ligament reconstruction. *Knee Surg Sports Traumatol Arthrosc.* 2017;25(2):493–500.
9. Cha PS, Brucker PU, West RV, et al. Arthroscopic double-bundle anterior cruciate ligament reconstruction: an anatomic approach. *Arthroscopy.* 2005;21(10):1275.
10. Irarrazaval S, Albers M, Chao T, Fu FH. Gross, arthroscopic, and radiographic anatomies of the anterior cruciate ligament: foundations for anterior cruciate ligament surgery. *Clin Sports Med.* 2017;36(1):9–23.
11. Lipscomb AB, Johnston RK, Snyder RB. The technique of cruciate ligament reconstruction. *Am J Sports Med.* 1981;9(2):77–81.
12. Schreiber VM, Jordan SS, Bonci GA, Irrgang JJ, Fu FH. The evolution of primary double-bundle ACL reconstruction and recovery of early post-operative range of motion. *Knee Surg Sports Traumatol Arthrosc.* 2017;25(5):1475–1481.
13. Gardner E, O'Rahilly R. The early development of the knee joint in staged human embryos. *J Anat.* 1968;102(Pt 2):289–299.
14. Haines RW. The early development of the femoro-tibial and tibio-fibular joints. *J Anat.* 1953;87(2):192–206.
15. Ratajczak W. Early development of the cruciate ligaments in staged human embryos. *Folia Morphol (Warsz).* 2000;59(4):285–290.
16. Merida-Velasco JA, Sanchez-Montesinos I, Espin-Ferra J, Merida-Velasco JR, Rodriguez-Vazquez JF, Jimenez-Collado J. Development of the human knee joint ligaments. *Anat Rec.* 1997;248(2):259–268.
17. Ferretti M, Levicoff EA, Macpherson TA, Moreland MS, Cohen M, Fu FH. The fetal anterior cruciate ligament: an anatomic and histologic study. *Arthroscopy.* 2007;23(3):278–283.
18. Tena-Arregui J, Barrio-Asensio C, Viejo-Tirado F, Puerta-Fonolla J, Murillo-Gonzalez J. Arthroscopic study of the knee joint in fetuses. *Arthroscopy.* 2003;19(8):862–868.
19. Matsumoto T, Ingham SM, Mifune Y, et al. Isolation and characterization of human anterior cruciate ligament-derived vascular stem cells. *Stem Cells Dev.* 2012;21(6):859–872.
20. Strocchi R, de Pasquale V, Gubellini P, et al. The human anterior cruciate ligament: histological and ultrastructural observations. *J Anat.* 1992;180(Pt 3):515–519.
21. Steckel H, Starman JS, Baums MH, Klinger HM, Schultz W, Fu FH. Anatomy of the anterior cruciate ligament double bundle structure: a macroscopic evaluation. *Scand J Med Sci Sports.* 2007;17(4):387–392.
22. Petersen W, Zantop T. Anatomy of the anterior cruciate ligament with regard to its two bundles. *Clin Orthop Relat Res.* 2007;454:35–47.
23. Zantop T, Petersen W, Sekiya JK, Musahl V, Fu FH. Anterior cruciate ligament anatomy and function relating to anatomical reconstruction. *Knee Surg Sports Traumatol Arthrosc.* 2006;14(10):982–992.
24. Giuliani JR, Kilcoyne KG, Rue JP. Anterior cruciate ligament anatomy: a review of the anteromedial and posterolateral bundles. *J Knee Surg.* 2009;22(2):148–154.
25. Kopf S, Pombo MW, Szczodry M, Irrgang JJ, Fu FH. Size variability of the human anterior cruciate ligament insertion sites. *Am J Sports Med.* 2011;39(1):108–113.
26. Steineman BD, Moulton SG, Donahue TLH, et al. Overlap between anterior cruciate ligament and anterolateral meniscal root insertions: a scanning electron microscopy study. *Am J Sports Med.* 2017;45(2):362–368.
27. Dienst M, Schneider G, Altmeyer K, et al. Correlation of intercondylar notch cross sections to the ACL size: a high resolution MR tomographic in vivo analysis. *Arch Orthop Trauma Surg.* 2007;127(4):253–260.
28. Wolters F, Vrooijink SH, Van Eck CF, Fu FH. Does notch size predict ACL insertion site size? *Knee Surg Sports Traumatol Arthrosc.* 2011;19(suppl 1):S17–S21.
29. Guenther D, Irarrazaval S, Albers M, et al. Area of the tibial insertion site of the anterior cruciate ligament as a predictor for graft size. *Knee Surg Sports Traumatol Arthrosc.* 2017;25(5):1576–1582.
30. Fujimaki Y, Thorhauer E, Sasaki Y, Smolinski P, Tashman S, Fu FH. Quantitative in situ analysis of the anterior cruciate ligament: length, midsubstance cross-sectional area, and insertion site areas. *Am J Sports Med.* 2016;44(1):118–125.
31. Ferretti M, Ekdahl M, Shen W, Fu FH. Osseous landmarks of the femoral attachment of the anterior cruciate ligament: an anatomic study. *Arthroscopy.* 2007;23(11):1218–1225.
32. Sasaki N, Ishibashi Y, Tsuda E, et al. The femoral insertion of the anterior cruciate ligament: discrepancy between macroscopic and histological observations. *Arthroscopy.* 2012;28(8):1135–1146.
33. Iwahashi T, Shino K, Nakata K, et al. Direct anterior cruciate ligament insertion to the femur assessed by histology and 3-dimensional volume-rendered computed tomography. *Arthroscopy.* 2010;26(suppl 9):S13–S20.
34. Haizuka Y, Nagase M, Takashino S, Kobayashi Y, Fujikura Y, Matsumura G. A new substitute for formalin: application to embalming cadavers. *Clin Anat.* 2018;31:90–98.
35. Steckel H, Vadala G, Davis D, Fu FH. 2D and 3D 3-tesla magnetic resonance imaging of the double bundle structure in anterior cruciate ligament anatomy. *Knee Surg Sports Traumatol Arthrosc.* 2006;14(11):1151–1158.
36. Steckel H, Vadala G, Davis D, Musahl V, Fu FH. 3-T MR imaging of partial ACL tears: a cadaver study. *Knee Surg Sports Traumatol Arthrosc.* 2007;15(9):1066–1071.
37. Katahira K, Yamashita Y, Takahashi M, et al. MR imaging of the anterior cruciate ligament: value of thin slice direct oblique coronal technique. *Radiat Med.* 2001;19(1):1–7.

38. Kosaka M, Nakase J, Toratani T, et al. Oblique coronal and oblique sagittal MRI for diagnosis of anterior cruciate ligament tears and evaluation of anterior cruciate ligament remnant tissue. *Knee*. 2014;21(1):54–57.

39. Kim SI, Park HJ, Lee SY, et al. Usefulness of oblique coronal and sagittal MR images of the knee after double-bundle and selective anterior cruciate ligament reconstructions. *Acta Radiol*. 2015;56(3):312–321.

40. Giugliano DN, Solomon JL. ACL tears in female athletes. *Phys Med Rehabil Clin N Am*. 2007;18(3):417–438. viii.

41. Toth AP, Cordasco FA. Anterior cruciate ligament injuries in the female athlete. *J Gender Specific Med*. 2001;4(4):25–34.

42. Sutton KM, Bullock JM. Anterior cruciate ligament rupture: differences between males and females. *Am Acad Orthop Surg*. 2013;21(1):41–50.

43. Sturnick DR, Vacek PM, DeSarno MJ, et al. Combined anatomic factors predicting risk of anterior cruciate ligament injury for males and females. *Am J Sports Med*. 2015;43(4):839–847.

44. Sturnick DR, Argentieri EC, Vacek PM, et al. A decreased volume of the medial tibial spine is associated with an increased risk of suffering an anterior cruciate ligament injury for males but not females. *J Orthop Res*. 2014;32(11):1451–1457.

45. Ireland ML. The female ACL: why is it more prone to injury? *Orthop Clin N Am*. 2002;33(4):637–651.

46. Anderson AF, Dome DC, Gautam S, Awh MH, Rennirt GW. Correlation of anthropometric measurements, strength, anterior cruciate ligament size, and intercondylar notch characteristics to sex differences in anterior cruciate ligament tear rates. *Am J Sports Med*. 2001;29(1):58–66.

47. Chandrashekar N, Slauterbeck J, Hashemi J. Sex-based differences in the anthropometric characteristics of the anterior cruciate ligament and its relation to intercondylar notch geometry: a cadaveric study. *Am J Sports Med*. 2005;33(10):1492–1498.

48. Muneta T, Takakuda K, Yamamoto H. Intercondylar notch width and its relation to the configuration and cross-sectional area of the anterior cruciate ligament. A cadaveric knee study. *Am J Sports Med*. 1997;25(1):69–72.

49. Miljko M, Grle M, Kozul S, Kolobaric M, Djak I. Intercondylar notch width and inner angle of lateral femoral condyle as the risk factors for anterior cruciate ligament injury in female handball players in Herzegovina. *Coll Antropol*. 2012;36(1):195–200.

50. Chandrashekar N, Mansouri H, Slauterbeck J, Hashemi J. Sex-based differences in the tensile properties of the human anterior cruciate ligament. *J Biomech*. 2006;39(16):2943–2950.

51. van Eck CF, Kopf S, van Dijk CN, Fu FH, Tashman S. Comparison of 3-dimensional notch volume between subjects with and subjects without anterior cruciate ligament rupture. *Arthroscopy*. 2011;27(9):1235–1241.

52. Griffin LY, Agel J, Albohm MJ, et al. Noncontact anterior cruciate ligament injuries: risk factors and prevention strategies. *J Am Acad Orthop Surg*. 2000;8(3):141–150.

CHAPTER 5

Anterior Cruciate Ligament Graft Choices in the Female Athlete

ARMANDO F. VIDAL, MD • CHRISTOPHER D. JOYCE, MD • MEREDITH MAYO, MD

INTRODUCTION

Although nonsurgical treatment of anterior cruciate ligament (ACL) ruptures is possible, the standard of care for young athletes is ACL reconstruction. A variety of grafts exist for ACL reconstruction in female athletes. In general, the grafts used for ACL reconstruction include autograft tissue, which is typically harvested from the ipsilateral limb, or cadaveric allograft tissue. The most commonly used autograft tissues include bone-patellar tendon-bone (BTB), hamstring tendon (HT), and quadriceps tendon (QT). Common allograft sources include BTB, Achilles tendon, QT, tibialis anterior tendon, tibialis posterior tendon, and HT. Choosing the correct graft for the correct patient is a highly debated topic across all patient populations and should be an individualized, patient-specific process. Several factors should be considered when choosing ACL grafts, including patient age, activity level, sport, concomitant injuries, gender, and surgeon's familiarity with the graft. While all these factors play a role for the female athlete, there is compelling evidence that well-performed surgeries with any graft type will produce good results.[1,2]

Graft choice for ACL reconstruction in female athletes requires particular scrutiny. Females undergoing ACL reconstruction have a lower rate of returning to sport than males.[3] One multicenter study found that 76% of male and 67% of female soccer athletes were able to return to playing soccer after ACL reconstruction.[4] When looking at success of the surgery, females were found to have an increased rate of revision surgery after ACL reconstruction. However, the graft failure rate was the same in both males and females. Females with an ACL rupture do have a significantly higher rate of contralateral ACL injuries than males, and they are roughly twice as likely to have a contralateral ACL rupture, as they are to fail their ACL reconstruction.[3,5]

It is important for practitioners and surgeons to inform female athlete patients about all the graft choices and the possible risks associated with surgery. This chapter highlights the most commonly utilized grafts for ACL reconstruction in the current orthopedic surgery community. While the choice of graft varies significantly from surgeon to surgeon, each graft does have certain advantages and disadvantages, which will be highlighted.

GRAFT OPTIONS

Bone-Patellar Tendon-Bone Autograft

One of the most commonly used autografts is the BTB autograft (Fig. 5.1). This graft has arguably the longest track record of use in orthopedic surgery and is widely considered to be the gold standard in ACL reconstruction.[6] The graft, as it is named, consists of a bone block at each of its end, with a slip of patellar tendon in between the two bone blocks. The slip of patellar tendon is typically the central one-third of the patellar tendon. The bone blocks are taken from the distal patella and the proximal tibial tubercle.

In our institution, the BTB autograft is harvested with a roughly 10-cm longitudinal incision over the medial border of the patellar tendon that also allows for final graft passage. The paratenon is incised, and the central third of the patellar tendon is measured and longitudinally incised, typically measuring 10 mm in width. An oscillating saw is used to resect a bone block out of the distal pole of the patella and the proximal portion of the tibial tubercle, and the graft is removed and prepared for passage into the corresponding femoral and tibial tunnels.

In addition to having a long and successful track record in ACL reconstruction, BTB grafts allow for bone-to-bone healing instead of soft tissue-to-bone incorporation. Biomechanical testing of BTB grafts demonstrates excellent tensile strength and increased load to failure (2900 N) when compared with the native ACL (1725 N) (Table 5.1).[7] The primary disadvantage with BTB autografts is donor site morbidity. Anterior knee pain and kneeling pain are the most common complaints, with up to 81% and 90% of patients, respectively, with such complaints in the first 2 years. Long-term follow-up, however, does show that

ACL Injuries in Female Athletes. https://doi.org/10.1016/B978-0-323-54839-7.00005-1

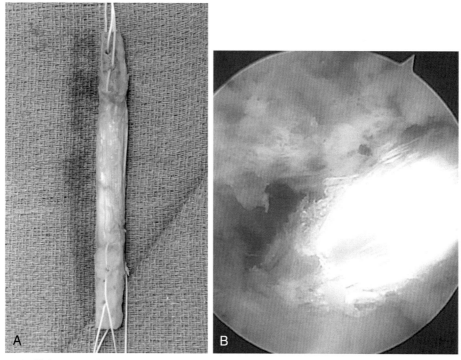

FIG. 5.1 **(A)** Intraoperative photograph showing a bone-patellar tendon-bone (BTB) autograft harvest, and **(B)** an arthroscopic photograph of a BTB graft placement.

TABLE 5.1
Average Loading Strengths of Each Graft Type

Graft Type	Load to Failure Strength (N)
Native anterior cruciate ligament	1725
Bone-patellar tendon-bone autograft	2900
Hamstring tendon autograft (quadrupled)	4090
Quadriceps tendon autograft	2352

these BTB harvest site issues are not significantly different from ACL reconstruction with HT autograft.[8] Less frequent causes of donor site morbidity include postoperative patella fracture and quadriceps weakness.[9–11]

No significant advantage in return to play or functional outcomes has been proven when comparing BTB autografts with other types of autografts.[12,13] A study by Gobbi et al. specifically compared BTB and HT autografts in male and female athletes and found that there were no significant differences between men and women in postoperative functional tests, laxity, or isokinetic exercises in patients with BTB autograft. The study did find that females with an HT autograft had increased laxity and a larger functional deficit in isokinetic exercises than males with HT autografts; however, no differences were found in direct comparison of BTB and HT autografts in the female group specifically.[14] Conversely, Kautzner et al.[11] compared ACL reconstruction with BTB and HT autografts in a randomized controlled fashion and found no significant functional or knee stability scores, but did find significantly more anterior knee pain in the BTB group.

There is no definitive data but BTB autografts may allow for better bony incorporation of the graft and less functional deficits than hamstring grafts; however, BTB autografts are also associated with more anterior knee pain, kneeling pain, and quadriceps weakness.

Hamstring Tendon Autograft
HT autografts along with BTB autografts comprise the majority of ACL autograft reconstructions (Fig. 5.2). Quadrupled HT autografts are the strongest autograft option available based on biomechanical testing, with

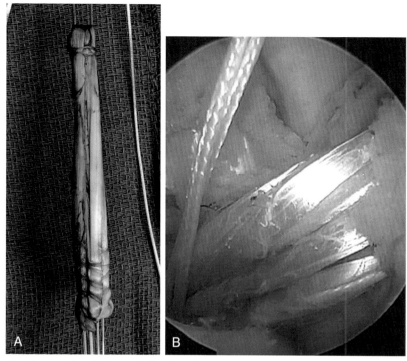

FIG. 5.2 **(A)** Intraoperative photograph showing a hamstring tendon (HT) autograft harvest, and **(B)** an arthroscopic photograph of an HT graft placement.

a maximal load to failure of 4090 N.[15] The graft is typically composed of a combination of the gracilis and semitendinosus tendons. The graft can be folded over, creating two- and four-strand HT autograft options. The graft has no bony blocks attached to it and relies on the tendon incorporating into the drill tunnel bone.

Our method of harvesting HT autograft starts with a longitudinal incision over the pes anserine insertion on the anteromedial proximal tibia, approximately midway between the tibial tubercle and the posteromedial border of the tibia. The sartorial fascia is incised carefully in an inverted "L" shape to protect the deeper medial collateral ligament. Invested within the sartorial fascia, the gracilis tendon insertion is identified proximally and isolated, while the semitendinosus tendon insertion is separated more distally. Under tension, each tendon is bluntly freed from frequently adherent deep fascial bridges to the medial gastrocnemius. Each tendon is carefully removed using a tendon stripper with slow force directed toward the muscular origins, as the gracilis originates from the inferior pubic ramus and the semitendinosus from the ischial tuberosity. The tendons are then folded and prepared for insertion.

In addition to their impressive strength, HT autografts result in less graft donor site morbidity, less short-term anterior knee pain, and less extensor lag when compared with BTB grafts.[16] The donor site morbidity associated with HT autograft does include some level of hamstring weakness.[17] Kim et al. found that HT autograft and allograft ACL reconstructions result in significantly decreased flexion strength compared with that of the contralateral uninjured limb. Those with HT autograft reconstruction had significantly weaker knee flexion (17.5% loss) than counterparts with allograft reconstruction (9.2% loss).[18] Whether this weakness is clinically relevant is another question, as it is not functionally limiting in most patients.

An important technical consideration for females is the diameter of the graft that is harvested from the gracilis and semitendinosus tendons. HT autografts with a diameter less than 8.0 mm are at an increased risk of failure compared with larger grafts.[19] Females, on average, have smaller-diameter HT grafts than males, with 42% of females having a graft diameter less than 7 mm.[20] This may place females at a theoretic increased risk of graft failure due to inherent smaller-diameter HT autografts. However, this result has not been shown in the literature. Another factor to consider is that females are relatively quadriceps dominant with weaker hamstrings when compared with males. This may contribute to a high rate of ACL injuries in female athletes, possibly increasing the risk of ACL reinjury after taking an HT autograft.[21] However, this is purely theoretic and has not been demonstrated clinically.

Quadriceps Tendon Autograft

The third most commonly used autograft is the QT autograft that is harvested as either a soft-tissue-only graft or a slip of central QT along with a single bone block from the patellar insertion. This type of autograft is not as frequently utilized in clinical practice. It does have similar donor site morbidity as a BTB graft, with anterior knee pain, risk of patella fractures, and quadriceps weakness. However, it also allows for bone-to-bone healing at one end of the graft. Clinical studies have varied, but for the most part, rerupture rate and clinical outcomes are similar for QT autografts when compared with BTB and HT grafts.[22,23] QT autografts are also a good option for revision ACL reconstruction, as they can be taken from the ipsilateral limb without interfering with the previous harvest sites at the knee. QT harvest does require a less cosmetically appealing incision on the thigh; however, this has improved with minimally invasive techniques.

Allograft

The first step in graft selection in a patient undergoing ACL reconstruction is deciding whether to use autograft or allograft tissue. Allograft tissue can be taken from several sources including BTB patellar tendon, Achilles tendon, tibialis posterior tendon, tibialis anterior tendon, peroneus longus tendon, and fascia lata. The primary advantage in using allograft is that it comes with no donor site morbidity. Patients do not have to worry about the anterior knee pain associated with BTB autografts or the hamstring weakness associated with hamstring autografts. Donor site morbidity is particularly important to consider in multiligamentous knee injury, as autograft reconstruction could contribute to further postoperative pain, weakness, and stiffness. Lastly, the use of allograft tissue does decrease operative time, as there is no graft harvest step.

In adolescents and skeletally immature patients, allograft ACL reconstructions have a significantly higher failure rate than autograft tissue. The failure rate of allograft ACL reconstructions in adolescents has been shown to be as high as 29%.[24,25] However, this trend has not been found in the adult population, with relatively equivalent functional results and failure rates between allografts and autografts in adults undergoing ACL reconstruction.[26] Allograft reconstructions also have a higher failure rate in the more active populations, with a failure rate of 44% found in a cohort of military recruits.[27]

Although allograft usage in female athletes has not been specifically studied, we do not recommend allograft use in any young athlete owing to the high risk of failure in this patient population. There may be a role for allograft ACL reconstruction in the middle-aged, recreational athlete, but any elite-level athlete or adolescent/pediatric patient would likely benefit from autograft reconstruction over allograft reconstruction.

Hybrid Hamstring Grafts

When an HT autograft is harvested and the diameter is inadequate (frequently considered as less than 7 mm), the graft may be augmented with allograft by creating a hybrid type graft. Hybrid hamstring grafts have a mixed success rate in the literature, with the majority of the evidence coming from retrospective reviews. Some studies demonstrated improved rerupture rates when compared with smaller hamstring autografts, whereas other studies showed no difference in rerupture rates or even higher rates of rerupture.[28–31] Based on current studies, the utility of hybrid HT grafts remains uncertain. Further studies are necessary to define their role as a potential option for adolescent females with small-diameter HTs (Table 5.2).

CONCLUSIONS AND RECOMMENDATIONS

ACL reconstruction in female athletes can be challenging, as this patient population is at a particularly high risk of recurrent injuries and graft failure. A myriad of options exist for graft choice in ACL reconstruction. Our recommendations for female athletes are to avoid allografts all together, if possible. We believe that QT autografts are a good option for revision scenarios, but long-term results from primary ACL reconstruction are not well elucidated. Female athletes function well with both HT and patellar tendon autografts, and the graft choice should be made on a case-by-case basis for the aforementioned reasons.

TABLE 5.2
Summary of the Advantages and Disadvantages of Each Graft Type

Graft Type	Advantages	Disadvantages
Bone-patellar tendon-bone autograft	• Bone-to-bone healing • Fastest biologic incorporation • Longest track record	• Anterior knee pain • Potential patella fracture
Hamstring tendon autograft	• Most cosmetic autograft • Highest graft strength	• Hamstring weakness • No bone-to-bone healing • Higher failure rate in small-diameter grafts
Quadriceps tendon autograft	• Bone-to-bone healing on one end of graft	• Less cosmetic incision • Anterior knee pain • Potential patella fracture
Allograft	• No donor site morbidity	• Highest failure rate

REFERENCES

1. Howard JS, Lembach ML, Metzler AV, Johnson DL. Rates and determinants of return to play after anterior cruciate ligament reconstruction in National Collegiate Athletic Association Division I soccer athletes: a study of the southeastern conference. *Am J Sports Med.* 2016;44(2):433–439. https://doi.org/10.1177/0363546515614315.
2. Allen MM, Pareek A, Krych AJ, et al. Are female soccer players at an increased risk of second anterior cruciate ligament injury compared with their athletic peers? *Am J Sports Med.* 2016;44(10):2492–2498. https://doi.org/10.1177/0363546516648439.
3. Tan SHS, Lau BPH, Khin LW, Lingaraj K. The importance of patient sex in the outcomes of anterior cruciate ligament reconstructions: a systematic review and meta-analysis. *Am J Sports Med.* 2016;44(1):242–254. https://doi.org/10.1177/0363546515573008.
4. Brophy RH, Schmitz L, Wright RW, et al. Return to play and future ACL injury risk after ACL reconstruction in soccer athletes from the Multicenter Orthopaedic Outcomes Network (MOON) group. *Am J Sports Med.* 2012;40(11):2517–2522. https://doi.org/10.1177/0363546512459476.
5. Paterno MV, Rauh MJ, Schmitt LC, Ford KR, Hewett TE. Incidence of second ACL injuries 2 years after primary ACL reconstruction and return to sport. *Am J Sports Med.* 2014;42(7):1567–1573. https://doi.org/10.1177/0363546514530088.
6. Duchman KR, Lynch TS, Spindler KP. Graft selection in anterior cruciate ligament surgery. *Clin Sports Med.* 2017;36(1):25–33. https://doi.org/10.1016/j.csm.2016.08.013.
7. Noyes FR, Butler DL, Grood ES, Zernicke RF, Hefzy MS. Biomechanical analysis of human ligament grafts used in knee-ligament repairs and reconstructions. *J Bone Joint Surg Am.* 1984;66(3):344–352. http://www.ncbi.nlm.nih.gov/pubmed/6699049.
8. Webster KE, Feller JA, Hartnett N, Leigh WB, Richmond AK. Comparison of patellar tendon and hamstring tendon anterior cruciate ligament reconstruction: a 15-year follow-up of a randomized controlled trial. *Am J Sports Med.* 2016;44(1):83–90. https://doi.org/10.1177/0363546515611886.
9. Rosenthal MD, Moore JH, Stoneman PD, DeBerardino TM. Neuromuscular excitability changes in the vastus medialis following anterior cruciate ligament reconstruction. *Electromyogr Clin Neurophysiol.* 2009;49(1):43–51. http://www.ncbi.nlm.nih.gov/pubmed/19280799.
10. Hiemstra LA, Webber S, Macdonald PB, Kriellaars DJ. Knee strength deficits after hamstring tendon and patellar tendon anterior cruciate ligament reconstruction. *Med Sci Sport Exerc.* 2000;32(8):1472–1479. https://doi.org/10.1097/00005768-200008000-00016.
11. Kautzner J, Kos P, Hanus M, Trc T, Havlas V. A comparison of ACL reconstruction using patellar tendon versus hamstring autograft in female patients: a prospective randomised study. *Int Orthop.* 2015;39(1):125–130. https://doi.org/10.1007/s00264-014-2495-7.
12. Kaeding CC, Pedroza AD, Reinke EK, et al. Risk factors and predictors of subsequent ACL injury in either knee after ACL reconstruction: prospective analysis of 2488 primary ACL reconstructions from the MOON cohort. *Am J Sports Med.* 2015;43(7):1583–1590. https://doi.org/10.1177/0363546515578836.
13. Mohtadi NG, Chan DS, Dainty KN, Whelan DB. Patellar tendon versus hamstring tendon autograft for anterior cruciate ligament rupture in adults. Chan DS, ed. *Cochrane Database Syst Rev.* 2011;(9):CD005960. https://doi.org/10.1002/14651858.CD005960.pub2.
14. Gobbi A, Domzalski M, Pascual J. Comparison of anterior cruciate ligament reconstruction in male and female athletes using the patellar tendon and hamstring autografts. *Knee Surgery, Sport Traumatol Arthrosc.* 2004;12(6):534–539. https://doi.org/10.1007/s00167-003-0486-0.

15. Hamner DL, Brown CH, Steiner ME, Hecker AT, Hayes WC. Hamstring tendon grafts for reconstruction of the anterior cruciate ligament: biomechanical evaluation of the use of multiple strands and tensioning techniques. *J Bone Joint Surg Am.* 1999;81(4):549–557. http://www.ncbi.nlm.nih.gov/pubmed/10225801.

16. Feller JA, Webster KE. A randomized comparison of patellar tendon and hamstring tendon anterior cruciate ligament reconstruction. *Am J Sports Med.* 2003;31(4):564–573. https://doi.org/10.1177/03635465030310041501.

17. Briem K, Ragnarsdóttir AM, Árnason SI, Sveinsson T. Altered medial versus lateral hamstring muscle activity during hop testing in female athletes 1-6 years after anterior cruciate ligament reconstruction. *Knee Surg Sports Traumatol Arthrosc.* 2016;24(1):12–17. https://doi.org/10.1007/s00167-014-3333-6.

18. Kim JG, Yang SJ, Lee YS, Shim JC, Ra HJ, Choi JY. The effects of hamstring harvesting on outcomes in anterior cruciate ligament-reconstructed patients: a comparative study between hamstring-harvested and -unharvested patients. *Arthroscopy.* 2011;27(9):1226–1234. https://doi.org/10.1016/j.arthro.2011.05.009.

19. Park SY, Oh H, Park S, Lee JH, Lee SH, Yoon KH. Factors predicting hamstring tendon autograft diameters and resulting failure rates after anterior cruciate ligament reconstruction. *Knee Surg Sports Traumatol Arthrosc.* 2013;21(5):1111–1118. https://doi.org/10.1007/s00167-012-2085-4.

20. Ma CB, Keifa E, Dunn W, Fu FH, Harner CD. Can preoperative measures predict quadruple hamstring graft diameter? *Knee.* 2010;17(1):81–83. https://doi.org/10.1016/j.knee.2009.06.005.

21. Myer GD, Ford KR, Barber Foss KD, Liu C, Nick TG, Hewett TE. The relationship of hamstrings and quadriceps strength to anterior cruciate ligament injury in female athletes. *Clin J Sport Med.* 2009;19(1):3–8. https://doi.org/10.1097/JSM.0b013e3181 90bddb.

22. Cavaignac E, Md Y, Coulin B, et al. Is quadriceps tendon autograft a better choice than hamstring autograft for anterior cruciate ligament reconstruction? A comparative study with a mean follow-up of 3.6 years. *Am J Sports Med.* 2017. https://doi.org/10.1177/0363546516688665.

23. Iriuchishima T, Ryu K, Okano T, Suruga M, Aizawa S, Fu FH. The evaluation of muscle recovery after anatomical single-bundle ACL reconstruction using a quadriceps autograft. *Knee Surgery Sport Traumatol Arthrosc.* 2017;25(5):1449–1453. https://doi.org/10.1007/s00167-016-4124-z.

24. Engelman GH, Carry PM, Hitt KG, Polousky JD, Vidal AF. Comparison of allograft versus autograft anterior cruciate ligament reconstruction graft survival in an active adolescent cohort. *Am J Sports Med.* 2014;42(10):2311–2318. https://doi.org/10.1177/0363546514541935.

25. Nelson IR, Chen J, Love R, Davis BR, Maletis GB, Funahashi TT. A comparison of revision and rerupture rates of ACL reconstruction between autografts and allografts in the skeletally immature. *Knee Surg Sport Traumatol Arthrosc.* 2016;24(3):773–779. https://doi.org/10.1007/s00167-016-4020-6.

26. Wei J, Yang H, Qin J, Yang T. A meta-analysis of anterior cruciate ligament reconstruction with autograft compared with nonirradiated allograft. *Knee.* 2015;22(5):372–379. https://doi.org/10.1016/j.knee.2014.06.006.

27. Pallis M, Svoboda SJ, Cameron KL, Owens BD. Survival comparison of allograft and autograft anterior cruciate ligament reconstruction at the United States Military Academy. *Am J Sports Med.* 2012;40(6):1242–1246. https://doi.org/10.1177/0363546512443945.

28. Jacobs CA, Burnham JM, Makhni EC, Malempati CS, Swart EC, Johnson DL. Allograft augmentation of hamstring autograft for younger patients undergoing anterior cruciate ligament reconstruction: clinical and cost-effectiveness analyses. *Am J Sports Med.* 2017;45(4):892–899. https://doi.org/10.1177/0363546516676079.

29. Darnley JE, Léger-St-Jean B, Pedroza AD, Flanigan DC, Kaeding CC, Magnussen RA. Anterior cruciate ligament reconstruction using a combination of autograft and allograft tendon. *Orthop J Sport Med.* 2016;4(7):232596711666224. https://doi.org/10.1177/2325967116662249.

30. Pennock AT, Ho B, Parvanta K, et al. Does allograft augmentation of small-diameter hamstring autograft ACL grafts reduce the incidence of graft retear? *Am J Sports Med.* 2017;45(2):334–338. https://doi.org/10.1177/0363546516677545.

31. Li J, Wang J, Li Y, Shao D, You X, Shen Y. A prospective randomized study of anterior cruciate ligament reconstruction with autograft, γ-irradiated allograft, and hybrid graft. *Arthrosc J Arthrosc Relat Surg.* 2015;31(7):1296–1302. https://doi.org/10.1016/j.arthro.2015.02.033.

CHAPTER 6

The Biology of Anterior Cruciate Ligament Healing After Reconstruction

ANDREA M. SPIKER, MD • SCOTT A. RODEO, MD

INTRODUCTION

Anterior cruciate ligament (ACL) rupture has become a common injury in the young, athletic population. As the number of young athletes continues to grow, an emphasis on sports specialization has led to increasing numbers of lower-extremity injuries,[1] including injuries such as ACL rupture. Reconstruction of the ACL has subsequently become a common orthopedic sports medicine surgical procedure that is performed with the goal of restoring stability to the knee and preventing further damage to cartilage and menisci. Recurrent ACL injury due to rupture of the ACL graft can be devastating. Younger athletes (aged <20 years) appear to have both a higher incidence of graft rupture and contralateral ACL injury after ACL reconstruction.[2] The rate of injury to the contralateral normal ACL appears to be at least the same, if not higher, as the rate of ACL graft rupture.[3] Understanding the biology of graft healing can provide insight into factors that affect healing and the risk of graft rupture.

A greater understanding of how and when graft healing occurs can also help to inform the design of a scientific rehabilitation program after ACL reconstruction. Rehabilitation guidelines after ACL reconstruction continue to evolve and should be based on the balance between protecting the graft in the healing process and maximizing the patient's return to functional and athletic ability. We have begun to realize that many athletes return to knee-strenuous sports earlier than they should, with persistent deficits in muscle function, coordination, proprioception, and balance,[4] but less is known about how our rehabilitation protocols correspond with the ACL graft healing process. The development of appropriate models to study the effect of postoperative mechanical loads on the healing graft will provide important insight into the design of postoperative rehabilitation programs and will help us to determine how and when patients should return to high-level athletic activities.[5–7]

Healing after ACL reconstruction is dependent on a number of factors, including graft type, surgical technique and strength of fixation, biomechanical and physiologic demands placed on the reconstruction, and the overall "biological milieu" of the knee. Biomechanical studies have demonstrated that the graft tissue itself (whether its autograft or allograft) is actually stronger than the native ACL at the time of implantation ("time zero").[8,9] This means that the femoral and tibial fixation points of the graft become the most important factors in determining whether or not the reconstruction fails in the early postoperative period.[10] The intra-articular portion of the tendon graft must undergo remodeling to become more like the original ligament, which occurs over a period after ACL reconstruction. The graft-to-bone attachment site in the tunnel is critical to ACL graft function, and thus healing at this interface is most important in the immediate postsurgical phase. In bone-containing grafts (bone-patella-bone or quadriceps tendon), bone-to-bone healing occurs with very strong biomechanical properties that are superior to those of soft tissue-to-bone healing.[11,12] With all-soft-tissue grafts (hamstring tendon), tendon-to-bone healing is required. It is prudent to note that all types of fibrous connective tissue (ligaments, tendons, etc.) attach to the bone surface in the human body, and the tendon inside a bone (a bone tunnel) is not seen anywhere in normal human anatomy. Even in bone-containing grafts a certain amount of tendon is required to heal the bone tunnel, as the graft is often recessed into the tunnel. There is evidence that several biological processes, such as macrophage-related inflammatory responses, expression of matrix metalloproteinases, and the presence of reactive oxygen species, can negatively impact the successful healing of the ACL graft.[13]

Further studies are clearly necessary to define the cellular and molecular mechanism(s) of ACL graft incorporation, graft healing, and eventual ACL graft function. This chapter will discuss our current understanding of the biology of ACL graft healing. A thorough understanding of this process can help in the design of scientific postoperative rehabilitation programs and provide insight into methods to improve graft healing, with the ultimate goal of optimizing patient outcomes after this common reconstructive surgery.

ACL Injuries in Female Athletes. https://doi.org/10.1016/B978-0-323-54839-7.00006-3

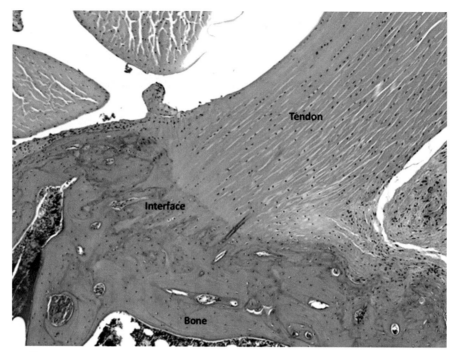

FIG. 6.1 Photomicrograph of normal anterior cruciate ligament insertion site. The tendon-to-bone interface is made up of unmineralized fibrocartilage and mineralized fibrocartilage (Scott Rodeo, 2018).

THE BIOLOGY OF THE NATIVE ANTERIOR CRUCIATE LIGAMENT

The function of the native ACL is to control rotational movements and the anterior translation of the tibia in relationship to the femur. It is an intra-articular extrasynovial structure made up of multiple collagen bundles. The major blood supply is from the middle genicular artery, and nerve innervation is from the tibial nerve, providing mostly vasomotor function, but some suggest a proprioceptive or sensory function. The complex multifascicular structure of the ACL allows different portions of the ligament to tense and function throughout full knee range of motion.[14]

The insertion site of the ligament to bone (at the femur and tibia) functions to diminish the stress concentration at the soft tissue-to-bone interface via a transition of unmineralized fibrocartilage and mineralized fibrocartilage. This type of transition is characteristic of a direct insertion site. Four distinct transition zones have been identified in the direct insertion fibers of the ACL: ligament, unmineralized fibrocartilage, mineralized fibrocartilage, and bone (Fig. 6.1). This gradual increase in structural stiffness allows for the efficient transfer of mechanical loads while minimizing peak stresses.[14–17] Collagen type X plays an important role

in the transition between the unmineralized and mineralized portion of the ligament insertion, but collagen types II, IX, and XI are also present. This suggests that the transition zone between bone and ligament is cartilaginous in nature.[16,17]

ACL reconstruction utilizing graft material does not recreate the microscopic structure and composition of the native ACL direct ligament enthesis. Instead, fibrovascular scar tissue forms at the graft-tunnel interface.[18,19] The attachment site between an ACL graft and bone resembles an indirect insertion, which consists of collagen fibers ("Sharpey fibers") anchoring into bone without a transitional zone of fibrocartilage. This healing graft-bone interface likely has inferior material properties, contributing to potential for micromotion at the graft-bone interface and risk of recurrent knee laxity (Fig. 6.2).

TIMELINE OF HEALING AFTER ANTERIOR CRUCIATE LIGAMENT RECONSTRUCTION

The following timeline of the microscopic events in ACL autograft healing is based on ACL reconstruction in animal models. Animal models have limitations in replicating the human postoperative state. It is difficult to stabilize the animal knee after ACL reconstruction,

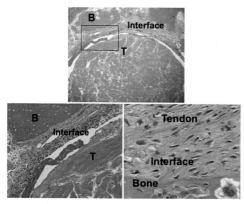

FIG. 6.2 Healing of a tendon graft in a bone tunnel occurs by the formation of a fibrovascular granulation tissue, with eventual formation of a "scar" tissue interface. There is establishment of collagen fiber continuity between the bone tunnel and the outer tendon, but the microscopic structure and composition of the native insertion site is not reformed. *B*, bone; *T*, tendon. (From Scott A. Rodeo, MD, Hospital for Special Surgery, New York, NY, USA.)

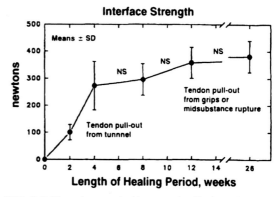

FIG. 6.3 There is a gradual increase in attachment strength of the healing tendon-bone interface over time. *NS*, not significant. (From Rodeo SA, Arnoczky SP, Torzilli PA, Hidaka C, Warren RF. Tendon-healing in a bone tunnel. A biomechanical and histological study in the dog. *J Bone Joint Surg Am.* 1993;75:1795–1803.)

which can result in ACL graft laxity. Attempts have been made with new animal models to overcome this limitation by minimizing postoperative mechanical loading of the graft. This can be accomplished with botulinum toxin and external fixation to temporarily limit excessive knee motion in order to evaluate the effect of mechanical load on ACL graft healing and incorporation.[5]

One to Two Weeks After Reconstruction

At 2 weeks after ACL reconstruction, osseous remodeling is noted at the edges of the bone tunnels, with both osteoclastic and osteoblastic activity. Tendinous grafts are surrounded by granulation tissue that forms in the interface between the graft and metaphyseal bone. The fibrovascular interface tissue likely contains pluripotent mesenchymal cells of bone marrow origin. Cells derived from synovium and synovial fluid may also participate in the early healing process. There is also ingrowth of capillaries and an influx of macrophages and fibroblasts.[19,20]

Three to Four Weeks After Reconstruction

At 3 weeks the granulation tissue surrounding the tendinous graft matures and begins to develop perpendicular collagen fibers extending to the bone tunnel, very similar to Sharpey fibers.[19] The mechanism of this maturation likely involves granulation tissue removal by macrophages.[20] New osteoid is seen at the edges of the bone tunnels. At this time point, the failure location of

tendinous grafts begins to change from pullout from the bone to failure through the intra-articular segment of the graft.[19] It is during the first 4 weeks that the greatest increases in interface strength are seen (Fig. 6.3).[20]

At 4 weeks, cells in the central portion of the graft are necrotic (with presence of pyknotic nuclei and ghost cells) but the matrix retains intact collagen fibers. There is a gradual increase in maturation and organization of collagen fibers between the bone tunnel and the graft.[19,21]

Six to Eight Weeks After Reconstruction

At 6 weeks, there is a more organized fibrovascular interface between the bone and graft. Immature fibroblasts, mononuclear cells, and macrophages are the predominant cell types in the healing interface at this time.[19] Between the 4- and 12-week mark, there is gradual cellular repopulation of the acellular portions of the intra-articular graft segment.[22–24]

Ten to Twelve Weeks After Reconstruction

At 12 weeks the tendon grafts demonstrate mature fibroblasts in the tissue surrounding the graft and the connective tissue is organized in a lamellar fashion.[19] The perpendicularly oriented collagen fibers are now circumferential around the graft.[18] The bone-soft tissue interface is now more continuous without a distinct differentiation.[19] After 12 weeks, graft failure during mechanical testing typically occurs because of intrasubstance graft failure or tendon avulsion from the edge of the bone tunnel, in contrast to early time points where graft failure occurs via tendon pullout from the bone tunnel.[18,20]

Nine Months After Reconstruction

At 9 months, graft revascularization and cellular repopulation results in the intra-articular portion of the graft beginning to resemble the native ligament on a microscopic level.[22-24]

Allograft Tendon Healing

Allograft tendon grafts appear to heal in a similar method to autograft, though the process is delayed compared with autograft tissue. The acellular graft tissue is replaced by host cells over time.[25] In an animal model, host DNA was found to have completely replaced donor allograft DNA in the intra-articular portion of the tendon graft by 4 weeks.[26] Angiogenesis, synovial cell and fibroblast infiltration, and matrix remodeling occur in a similar method as described for autograft. Animal studies suggest that allograft tendons may lose more of their initial tensile strength than autograft tendons during the graft incorporation and remodeling process, which may have important implications for the postoperative rehabilitation of patients who have allograft ACL reconstruction.[26]

Another consideration in allograft tendon healing is the effect of graft processing and sterilization. Allograft tissue can be subjected to chemicals, deep freezing, or radiation to decrease the risk of bacterial contamination and transmission of infectious diseases. Each of these methods attempts to decrease the risk of transmission of bacterial or viral pathogens.

Allograft tissue may also invoke an immune response, which may affect the process of graft incorporation and remodeling. Graft processing techniques may decrease but not completely eliminate immunogenicity of the graft tissue. Chemical sterilization is thought to be the most detrimental for allograft tendons, as it may lead to a heightened inflammatory reaction and adversely affect graft material properties, resulting in decreased strength and delayed remodeling. Deep freezing the allografts may not completely denature cell surface human leukocyte antigens in the donor tissue, resulting in a persistent risk of a host immune response directed against the graft.[27] γ-Irradiated grafts demonstrate diminished strength in the controlled laboratory setting and an increased rate of failure in the clinical setting when compared with autografts or fresh frozen allografts.[28,29] Different doses of γ-radiation are required to eradicate various pathogens: 0.5 mRad of radiation will eliminate non-spore-forming bacteria, whereas up to 2.1 Mrad is required for spore-forming bacteria. Doses of 0.8 Mrad are required for yeasts and molds, and HIV eradication can require between 1.5 and 4.0 Mrad.[30] Most believe

that lower doses of radiation (1.0–2.0 Mrad) will not affect the biomechanical properties of an allograft[30]; however, one study reported an 8.8% failure rate and a higher incidence of recurrent laxity with a dose of 1.5–2.5 mRad of radiation.[28] These lower doses will also fail to eradicate spore-forming bacteria, HIV, and hepatitis virus, so additional extensive screening is required.[30]

THE EFFECT OF BIOMECHANICAL LOADS ON GRAFT HEALING

The strength of the graft-to-bone tunnel interface achieves the most gains during the first 4 weeks after ACL reconstruction. Animal models suggest that the mode of graft failure changes from pullout at the tendon-bone interface to failure at the graft midsubstance between 8 and 12 weeks postoperatively.[20] The question of how variation in biomechanical loads across this interface affects the biological events in graft incorporation is very clinically relevant, as it translates into how we rehabilitate patients postoperatively to achieve the fastest return to activities and sports without compromising the ACL graft healing.

Excessive loads on the healing graft in the early postoperative period can result in micromotion at the graft-to-bone interface, which can lead to a sustained inflammatory response that is detrimental to continued healing. Osteoclast activation can also occur, resulting in bone resorption and tunnel widening.[31-33] Patients subjected to rehabilitation protocols with early motion were noted to have significant increases in tibial tunnel widening within the first 3 months after surgery.[31] In general, slower healing is noted at tunnel apertures where tunnel-graft motion is the highest.[20] Animal studies demonstrate that delayed application of cyclic axial loads (after a period of immobilization) results in superior tendon-to-bone healing by both biological and biomechanical parameters when compared with immediate loading or loading after a prolonged period of immobilization.[34,35]

FACTORS THAT NEGATIVELY AFFECT ANTERIOR CRUCIATE LIGAMENT GRAFT HEALING

Much of what we know about the factors that negatively impact the healing process is based on studies of primary repair after ACL rupture. While a new technique for primary ACL repair with biological scaffold reinforcement has been described and is in the very early stages of clinical trials,[36,37] classic studies described a 20%–40% complete failure rate of primary ACL repair,[38] with as many as 94% of patients demonstrating instability at 5 years.[39] The biological milieu of the intra-articular environment after ACL rupture is quite different than that of extra-articular injuries, such as the medial collateral ligament. The intra-articular environment demonstrates an increase in the level of inflammatory mediators and matrix-degrading enzymes (matrix metalloproteinases), which can adversely affect graft healing and remodeling. There is also a decreased concentration of some cytokines that are felt to play an important role in the healing response, such as fibrinogen, platelet-derived growth factor, transforming growth factor β, and fibroblast growth factor. This results in diminished ability of the ACL to heal primarily[40] and may play a role in inhibiting or delaying ACL graft healing as well.

AVENUES TO IMPROVE HEALING POTENTIAL AFTER ACL RECONSTRUCTION

Further knowledge about the factors that negatively affect ACL graft healing can aide in the development of techniques to improve outcomes after reconstruction. Technical modifications, biological augmentations, and changes in postoperative rehabilitation have all been attempted.

Technical modifications to increase the bone tunnel length, tighten the graft fit within the tunnel, and create circumferential contact of the graft to bone tunnel (by eliminating an interference screw) have all shown promise in improving graft healing in animal studies.[41–43] However, there is currently very little clinical data available to support the role of these techniques.

At the cellular and molecular levels the inflammatory response appears to play a fundamental role in the successful integration of the graft to native bone. A number of inflammatory cell types and inflammatory mediators are expressed and active during various phases of the graft healing process. Cyclooxygenase (COX) enzymes appear to play a role in the early tendon-to-bone healing process. Studies have shown that COX-2 inhibitors and other nonsteroidal anti-inflammatory drugs (NSAIDs) can impair bony integration of the graft.[44,45] In the animal model a significant decrease in bone healing was noted after 5 weeks of continuous COX-2 inhibition or ketorolac administration, and even 2 weeks of COX-2 inhibition resulted in significantly less new bone formation. Also in the animal model, local administration of prostaglandin E_2 leads to enhanced bone healing.[44] However, the clinical data on the effect of NSAIDs and COX-2 inhibitors on graft healing remain mixed, in large part owing to the lack of prospective randomized controlled trials addressing this question.[46,47]

Platelet-rich plasma (PRP) has been investigated for its potential role in stimulating healing after ACL reconstruction. Intra-articular use of PRP alone does not result in improved healing, as intra-articular plasmin breaks down the fibrin within PRP.[48] Several small studies have demonstrated a faster rate of graft maturation based on MRI after soaking the graft in PRP, but they have failed to show an improvement in patient-reported outcomes or evidence of improved healing.[49,50] Utilizing a collagen-based bioactive scaffold in combination with PRP is the basis of the ACL repair research by Murray et al. The scaffold may protect against the intra-articular degradation of plasmin and optimize the healing potential of PRP.[36,51,52] Studies focusing on the tunnel-graft interface have shown some promise in the animal model. Vogrin et al.[53] found that using PRP at the tunnel-graft interface increased vascularization at early time points (4–6 weeks) but not during the later healing process. In one study, application of bone marrow mesenchymal stem cells and vascular endothelial growth factor to the bone-tunnel interface showed improvement in healing in the animal model, which was determined by increased collagen type III, increased MRI signal intensity, and biomechanical tests of ultimate tensile strength.[54]

CONCLUSION

The biology of ACL graft healing is influenced by many different factors over an extended period of time, including the biomechanical loading of the graft and the biological milieu of the knee. As we gain a better understanding of the factors that both negatively and positively affect healing, we can continue to improve on our surgical and postoperative treatment of ACL reconstruction to optimize graft healing and patient outcomes.

REFERENCES

1. McGuine TA, et al. A prospective study on the effect of sport specialization on lower extremity injury rates in high school athletes. *Am J Sports Med*. 2017;45:2706–2712.
2. Webster KE, Feller JA, Leigh WB, Richmond AK. Younger patients are at increased risk for graft rupture and contralateral injury after anterior cruciate ligament reconstruction. *Am J Sports Med*. 2014;42:641–647.
3. Wright RW, Magnussen RA, Dunn WR, Spindler KP. Ipsilateral graft and contralateral ACL rupture at five years or more following ACL reconstruction. *J Bone Jt Surg*. 2011;93:1159–1165.

4. Beischer S, Senorski EH, Thomeé C, Samuelsson K, Thomeé R. Young athletes return too early to knee-strenuous sport, without acceptable knee function after anterior cruciate ligament reconstruction. *Knee Surgery Sport Traumatol Arthrosc.* 2017. https://doi.org/10.1007/s00167-017-4747-8.

5. Lebaschi A, et al. Restriction of postoperative Joint loading in a Murine model of anterior cruciate ligament reconstruction: botulinum toxin paralysis and external fixation. *J Knee Surg.* 2017;30:687–693.

6. Rodeo SA, et al. Use of a new model allowing controlled uniaxial loading to evaluate tendon healing in a bone tunnel. *J Orthop Res.* 2016;34:852–859.

7. Ma R, Ju X, Deng X-H, Rodeo S. A novel small animal model of differential anterior cruciate ligament reconstruction graft strain. *J Knee Surg.* 2014;28:489–495.

8. Hamner DL, Brown CH, Steiner ME, Hecker AT, Hayes WC. Hamstring tendon grafts for reconstruction of the anterior cruciate ligament: biomechanical evaluation of the use of multiple strands and tensioning techniques. *J Bone Joint Surg Am.* 1999;81:549–557.

9. Cooper DE, Deng XH, Burstein AL, Warren RF. The strength of the central third patellar tendon graft. A biomechanical study. *Am J Sports Med.* 1993;21:818–823; discussion 823–4.

10. Kurosaka M, Yoshiya S, Andrish JT. A biomechanical comparison of different surgical techniques of graft fixation in anterior cruciate ligament reconstruction. *Am J Sports Med.* 1987;15:225–229.

11. Papageorgiou CD, Ma CB, Abramowitch SD, Clineff TD, Woo SL. A multidisciplinary study of the healing of an intraarticular anterior cruciate ligament graft in a goat model. *Am J Sports Med.* 2001;29:620–626.

12. Tomita F, et al. Comparisons of intraosseous graft healing between the doubled flexor tendon graft and the bone-patellar tendon-bone graft in anterior cruciate ligament reconstruction. *Arthroscopy.* 2001;17:461–476.

13. Song B, et al. Macrophage M1 plays a positive role in aseptic inflammation-related graft loosening after anterior cruciate ligament reconstruction surgery. *Inflammation.* 2017;40:1815–1824.

14. Arnoczky SP. Anatomy of the anterior cruciate ligament. *Clin Orthop Relat Res.* 1983:19–25.

15. Sasaki N, et al. The femoral insertion of the anterior cruciate ligament: discrepancy between macroscopic and histological observations. *Arthroscopy.* 2012;28:1135–1146.

16. Fujioka H, et al. Comparison of surgically attached and non-attached repair of the rat Achilles tendon-bone interface. Cellular organization and type X collagen expression. *Connect Tissue Res.* 1998;37:205–218.

17. Niyibizi C, Sagarrigo Visconti C, Gibson G, Kavalkovich K. Identification and immunolocalization of type X collagen at the ligament-bone interface. *Biochem Biophys Res Commun.* 1996;222:584–589.

18. Goradia VK, Rochat MC, Grana WA, Rohrer MD, Prasad HS. Tendon-to-bone healing of a semitendinosus tendon autograft used for ACL reconstruction in a sheep model. *Am J Knee Surg.* 2000;13:143–151.

19. Grana WA, Egle DM, Mahnken R, Goodhart CW. An analysis of autograft fixation after anterior cruciate ligament reconstruction in a rabbit model. *Am J Sports Med.* 1994;22:344–351.

20. Rodeo SA, Arnoczky SP, Torzilli PA, Hidaka C, Warren RF. Tendon-healing in a bone tunnel. A biomechanical and histological study in the dog. *J Bone Joint Surg Am.* 1993;75:1795–1803.

21. Jackson DW, Simon TM. Donor cell survival and repopulation after intraarticular transplantation of tendon and ligament allografts. *Microsc Res Tech.* 2002;58:25–33.

22. Panni AS, Milano G, Lucania L, Fabbriciani C. Graft healing after anterior cruciate ligament reconstruction in rabbits. *Clin Orthop Relat Res.* 1997:203–212.

23. Kleiner JB, Amiel D, Roux RD, Akeson WH. Origin of replacement cells for the anterior cruciate ligament autograft. *J Orthop Res.* 1986;4:466–474.

24. Arnoczky SP, Tarvin GB, Marshall JL. Anterior cruciate ligament replacement using patellar tendon. An evaluation of graft revascularization in the dog. *J Bone Joint Surg Am.* 1982;64:217–224.

25. Min BH, Han MS, Woo JI, Park HJ, Park SR. The origin of cells that repopulate patellar tendons used for reconstructing anterior cruciate ligaments in man. *J Bone Joint Surg Br.* 2003;85:753–757.

26. Jackson DW, Corsetti J, Simon TM. Biologic incorporation of allograft anterior cruciate ligament replacements. *Clin Orthop Relat Res.* 1996:126–133.

27. Muller B, Bowman KF, Bedi A. ACL graft healing and biologics. *Clin Sports Med.* 2013;32:93–109.

28. Guo L, et al. Anterior cruciate ligament reconstruction with bone-patellar tendon-bone graft: comparison of autograft, fresh-frozen allograft, and γ-irradiated allograft. *Arthroscopy.* 2012;28:211–217.

29. Curran AR, Adams DJ, Gill JL, Steiner ME, Scheller AD. The biomechanical effects of low-dose irradiation on bone-patellar tendon-bone allografts. *Am J Sports Med.* 2004;32:1131–1135.

30. Yanke AB, et al. The biomechanical effects of 1.0 to 1.2 Mrad of gamma irradiation on human bone–patellar tendon–bone allografts. *Am J Sports Med.* 2013;41:835–840.

31. Hantes ME, Mastrokalos DS, Yu J, Paessler HH. The effect of early motion on tibial tunnel widening after anterior cruciate ligament replacement using hamstring tendon grafts. *Arthroscopy.* 2004;20:572–580.

32. Rodeo SA, Kawamura S, Kim H-J, Dynybil C, Ying L. Tendon healing in a bone tunnel differs at the tunnel entrance versus the tunnel exit: an effect of graft-tunnel motion? *Am J Sports Med.* 2006;34:1790–1800.

33. Ma R, et al. Effect of dynamic changes in anterior cruciate ligament in situ graft force on the biological healing response of the graft-tunnel interface. *Am J Sports Med.* 2018;46:915–923.

34. Bedi A, et al. Effect of early and delayed mechanical loading on tendon-to-bone healing after anterior cruciate ligament reconstruction. *J Bone Jt Surg Am.* 2010;92:2387–2401.

35. Camp CL, et al. Timing of postoperative mechanical loading affects healing following anterior cruciate ligament reconstruction. *J Bone Jt Surg*. 2017;99:1382–1391.

36. Murray MM, et al. The bridge-enhanced anterior cruciate ligament repair (BEAR) procedure. *Orthop J Sport Med*. 2016;4:232596711667217.

37. Perrone GS, et al. Bench-to-bedside: bridge-enhanced anterior cruciate ligament repair. *J Orthop Res*. 2017. https://doi.org/10.1002/jor.23632.

38. Marshall JL, Warren RF, Wickiewicz TL. Primary surgical treatment of anterior cruciate ligament lesions. *Am J Sports Med*. 1982;10:103–107.

39. Feagin JA, Curl WW. Isolated tear of the anterior cruciate ligament: 5-year followup study. *Clin Orthop Relat Res*. 1996:4–9.

40. Murray MM, Bennett R, Zhang X, Spector M. Cell outgrowth from the human ACL in vitro: regional variation and response to TGF-beta1. *J Orthop Res*. 2002;20:875–880.

41. Yamazaki S, Yasuda K, Tomita F, Minami A, Tohyama H. The effect of intraosseous graft length on tendon-bone healing in anterior cruciate ligament reconstruction using flexor tendon. *Knee Surg Sports Traumatol Arthrosc*. 2006;14:1086–1093.

42. Greis PE, Burks RT, Bachus K, Luker MG. The influence of tendon length and fit on the strength of a tendon-bone tunnel complex. A biomechanical and histologic study in the dog. *Am J Sports Med*. 2001;29:493–497.

43. Singhatat W, Lawhorn KW, Howell SM, Hull ML. How four weeks of implantation affect the strength and stiffness of a tendon graft in a bone tunnel: a study of two fixation devices in an extraarticular model in ovine. *Am J Sports Med*. 2002;30:506–513.

44. O'Keefe RJ, et al. COX-2 has a critical role during incorporation of structural bone allografts. *Ann N Y Acad Sci*. 2006;1068:532–542.

45. Sauerschnig M, et al. Effect of COX-2 inhibition on tendon-to-bone healing and PGE2 concentration after anterior cruciate ligament reconstruction. *Eur J Med Res*. 2018;23:1.

46. Pullen WM, et al. Predictors of revision surgery after anterior cruciate ligament reconstruction. *Am J Sports Med*. 2016;44:3140–3145.

47. Soreide E, et al. The effect of limited perioperative non-steroidal anti-inflammatory drugs on patients undergoing anterior cruciate ligament reconstruction. *Am J Sports Med*. 2016;44:3111–3118.

48. Figueroa D, et al. Platelet-rich plasma use in anterior cruciate ligament surgery: systematic review of the literature. *Arthrosc J Arthrosc Relat Surg*. 2015;31:981–988.

49. Figueroa D, et al. Magnetic resonance imaging evaluation of the integration and maturation of semitendinosus-gracilis graft in anterior cruciate ligament reconstruction using autologous platelet concentrate. *Arthroscopy*. 2010;26:1318–1325.

50. Nin JRV, Gasque GM, Azcárate AV, Beola JDA, Gonzalez MH. Has platelet-rich plasma any role in anterior cruciate ligament allograft healing? *Arthroscopy*. 2009;25:1206–1213.

51. Murray MM, et al. Collagen-platelet rich plasma hydrogel enhances primary repair of the porcine anterior cruciate ligament. *J Orthop Res*. 2007;25:81–91.

52. Murray MM, et al. Enhanced histologic repair in a central wound in the anterior cruciate ligament with a collagen-platelet-rich plasma scaffold. *J Orthop Res*. 2007;25:1007–1017.

53. Vogrin M, et al. Effects of a platelet gel on early graft revascularization after anterior cruciate ligament reconstruction: a prospective, randomized, double-blind, clinical trial. *Eur Surg Res*. 2010;45:77–85.

54. Setiawati R, Utomo DN, Rantam FA, Ifran NN, Budhiparama NC. Early graft tunnel healing after anterior cruciate ligament reconstruction with intratunnel injection of bone marrow mesenchymal stem cells and vascular endothelial growth factor. *Orthop J Sport Med*. 2017;5:232596711770854.

FURTHER READING

1. Gulotta LV, Rodeo SA. Biology of autograft and allograft healing in anterior cruciate ligament reconstruction. *Clin Sports Med*. 2007;26:509–524.

2. Quain J. In: Sharpey W, Ellis GV, eds. *Elements of Anatomy by Jones Quain*. 6th ed. vol. 1. London: Walton and Moberly; 1856.

CHAPTER 7

Special Considerations: Pediatric Anterior Cruciate Ligament

PAMELA J. LANG, MD • MININDER S. KOCHER, MD, MPH

INTRODUCTION

As the number of girls participating in organized sports has increased, so has the incidence of sports-related injuries. Likewise, the number of ACL injuries diagnosed in young athletes has increased. In a study of youth athletes, 47% of preadolescents and 65% of adolescents presenting with knee hemarthrosis after acute injury were ultimately found to have an ACL rupture.[1]

Gender differences in noncontact ACL injury have consistently been found.[2–8] Overall, the prevalence of noncontact ACL injuries in female athletes is approximately 10%–20% higher than that in male athletes.[2–5] In a study of collegiate athletes, female soccer and basketball players had 2.7 times higher incidence of ACL injury than their male counterparts.[3] In contrast, a study of injuries treated at a large academic children's hospital found that 10% of males and 8.9% of females were treated for an ACL tear,[9] suggesting that rates of ACL injury may be similar in younger children.

NONCONTACT ANTERIOR CRUCIATE LIGAMENT INJURIES IN FEMALE ATHLETES

During adolescence the overall and relative risk of ACL injury in females increases dramatically.[2–4,6,8–10] Genetic factors (familial predisposition, collagen polymorphisms), anatomic factors (narrow notch width, increased tibial slope), hormonal factors, and biomechanical/neuromuscular factors (decreased hip abduction strength, jump-landing mechanics) have been shown to be the risk factors for ACL injury.[11,12] Female athletes have been the subjects of several studies assessing factors associated with noncontact ACL injury.

Anatomic factors shown to be associated with ACL injury include increased posterior slope of the lateral tibial plateau and narrow intercondylar notch. The lateral tibial slope, as measured by MRI, has been found to be associated with ACL injury in pediatric and adolescent patients.[13,14] Beynnon et al.[14] evaluated and compared the lateral tibial slope in a cohort of individuals with a history of ACL injury and that in matched

controls. Each degree increase in the posterior tibial slope was associated with a 21.7% increase in the risk of ACL injury among females, but this was not found among males.[14] A narrow intercondylar notch has been shown to be associated with an increased risk of ACL injury.[15–18] Among skeletally immature individuals, a narrow intercondylar notch, as measured by notch width index, was associated with intrasubstance ACL tear rather than tibial spine avulsion.[15]

Given the sex differences in the incidence of ACL injury, which begins to emerge during adolescence, the impact of sex hormones on ACL injury risk has been studied.[12] Estrogen and progesterone, which vary in concentration throughout the menstrual cycle, have been found to have receptors on the ACL.[12] Studies have shown variable associations between ACL injury and the various phases of the menstrual cycle.[12] These analyses are difficult because techniques for measuring and categorizing the phase of the menstrual cycle are variable.

Biomechanical and neuromuscular factors for ACL injury have been studied. When evaluating jump-landing mechanics in males and females, kinetic and kinematic differences have been found between males and females, particularly during adolescence.[7,8] Hewett et al.[19] prospectively evaluated female high-school athletes and compared the biomechanical factors of those who sustained ACL injuries with those of athletes who did not. The observed biomechanical risk factors in the ACL-injured female athletes included increased knee valgus, decreased knee flexion, asymmetric landing from a drop vertical jump, and excessive ground reaction force.[19]

Neuromuscular control and trunk and hip strength have been shown to have an association with noncontact ACL injury.[20–22] In a 3-year prospective study, ACL injuries in female athletes were predicted with 91% accuracy using trunk displacements, proprioception, and a history of low-back pain as the indicators of future ACL injury.[21] The same model for predicting ACL injury was not applicable to male athletes.[21] Similarly, lateral trunk flexion and knee valgus angles, as measured by

ACL Injuries in Female Athletes. https://doi.org/10.1016/B978-0-323-54839-7.00007-5

video analysis of National Basketball Association and Women's National Basketball Association players, were significantly greater in female basketball players who sustained ACL injuries than in the male players and female players who did not injure their ACLs.[20] Furthermore, both hip abductor and external rotator weakness were significant neuromuscular risk factors for future noncontact ACL injury in males and females.[23]

MANAGEMENT OF ANTERIOR CRUCIATE LIGAMENT INJURIES IN PEDIATRIC PATIENTS

Treatment options for ACL injury are nonoperative management or operative reconstruction. Some patients with partial ACL injuries can be treated successfully with nonoperative management including bracing, physical therapy, and activity modification.[24] In contrast, nonoperative treatment of patients with complete ACL injuries has been shown to result in persistent instability and subsequent meniscal and chondral injuries.[25-30] In response to the increasing number of ACL injuries in young patients and the documented negative outcomes with nonoperative management, pediatric and adolescent ACL reconstruction techniques have gained popularity. The number of skeletally immature patients undergoing ACL reconstruction has increased dramatically over the past two decades. Between 1994 and 2006 the number of ACL reconstructions performed in patients younger than 15 years increased by 924%.[31]

Preoperative planning should consider the skeletal, physical, and psychologic maturity of the patient. The bone age should be evaluated using a single anteroposterior radiograft of the hand and wrist.[32] While evaluating physical maturity using Tanner stage may be difficult in an orthopedic clinic, a female patient's menstrual history can be helpful information. Additionally, at the time of clinical assessment, it is essential to discuss postoperative recovery and activity restrictions with patients and their families in order to set expectations.

An important consideration in ACL reconstruction is graft choice: autograft versus allograft. The Multicenter Orthopaedic Outcomes Network (MOON) study showed that the graft failure rate of allograft tissue in patients aged 10–19 years was four times greater than when autograft was used.[33] Therefore, autograft tissue should be considered the gold standard for ACL reconstruction in the young athlete.

ACL reconstruction techniques for pediatric patients include physeal sparing, physeal respecting, and transphyseal ACL reconstruction.[34-38] An algorithm for ACL reconstruction in young patients is presented in Fig. 7.1.

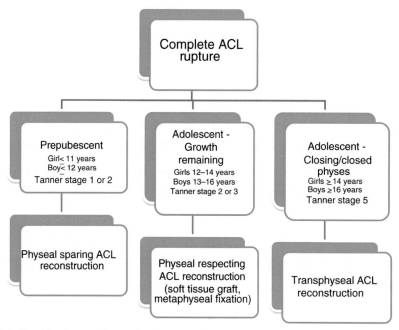

FIG. 7.1 Algorithm for anterior cruciate ligament (ACL) reconstruction in children and adolescents.

Two different physeal sparing ACL reconstruction techniques predominate: the intra-articular and extra-articular iliotibial band reconstruction, as described by Kocher and Micheli,[34,35] and the anatomic all-epiphyseal technique, as described by Anderson.[36] The physeal sparing intra-articular and extra-articular ACL reconstruction utilizing iliotibial band autograft has been shown to have a low failure rate (4.5%) with no reported growth disturbances.[34,35] The extra-articular component of this reconstruction simulates reconstruction of the anterolateral ligament, which in conjunction with the intra-articular ACL reconstruction may account for the low rate of graft failure in this technique. The all-epiphyseal ACL reconstruction can be technically demanding and graft fixation may be complicated by short or shallow tibial tunnels.[36] In a series of 103 patients who were treated with all-epiphyseal ACL reconstruction with hamstring autograft, graft retear rate was 10.7% and only one patient was found to have a leg length discrepancy (<1 cm).[38] During the follow-up period, 2.9% of the patients in that cohort had sustained subsequent meniscal tears.[38]

Adolescents with growth remaining may be candidates for physeal respecting ACL reconstruction. With physeal respecting ACL reconstruction, soft tissue grafts are utilized and fixation of the graft is positioned in the metaphysis, away from the physis. Animal studies have shown that soft tissue interposition at the site of physeal injury is protective against premature physeal closure.[39] It is also recommended that less than 7% of the physis be violated in order to prevent growth disturbance.[31] Therefore, femoral and tibial tunnels can be drilled slightly more vertically to produce a smaller zone of injury within the physis. Studies have shown good functional results and no growth disturbances using this physeal respecting technique in adolescent patients with growth remaining.[40,41] Despite the safety of this technique in respect to the potential for growth disturbance, the risk of graft tear in this group has been reported to be 11%, with a 24% incidence of reoperation.[40,42] The high risk of graft tear in this young population may be associated with return to high-risk activities in this population.

In contrast to the physeal sparing and physeal respecting ACL reconstruction techniques used in children and adolescents with growth remaining, the transphyseal technique, as performed in adults, may be used in skeletally mature and nearly mature adolescents. Transphyseal ACL reconstruction in skeletally mature and nearly mature individuals can utilize either a soft tissue graft or a graft with bone plugs without concern for location of fixation.

REHABILITATION

Adequate rehabilitation following ACL reconstruction may help athletes to regain adequate motion, strength, proprioception, and neuromuscular control to allow them to return to sports. For younger patients, it is ideal to have a therapist experienced in working with children and adolescents, as techniques to engage and motivate children may be different from those used in adults. Fostering compliance and self-directed activity can be a challenge in younger patients. Additionally, cues given to athletes during rehabilitation should be based on the developmental stages of children and adolescents.[43]

Early therapy following ACL reconstruction focuses on regaining range of motion, patellar mobilization, and muscle activation. Full extension, isometric strengthening, and early weight bearing are encouraged in the first 1–2 weeks following surgery.[44,45] Additionally, as patients reach early rehabilitative goals, closed chain strengthening exercises, balance, and neuromuscular retraining become the subsequent focus of rehabilitation. Jogging is generally allowed starting 3 months after surgery with progressioin to plyometric and more sport-specific exercises by 6 months postoperatively.

RETURN TO SPORTS

According to a report, 96% of young patients (<14 years) return to sports at the same level following ACL reconstruction.[46] In a retrospective review of skeletally immature patients, the median time for return to sport was 9 months and 85% were able to return to sports at 1 year.[46]

The criteria for determining readiness for return to play after ACL reconstruction are not well understood or agreed upon. More objective criteria have been employed to determine when an athlete is ready to return to sport. The Limb Symmetry Index (LSI) reports the relative performance of the operative limb in comparison to the uninjured limb.[44] The LSI should take into consideration a diverse battery of functional tests including strength tests, balance tests, hop tests, and agility tests.[44] An LSI of >90% has been used to suggest safe return to sports. Some even suggest that an LSI of 100% be reached prior to return to cutting and pivoting sports.[44] In addition to LSI, the ratio of hamstrings to quadriceps strength has been shown to be an important consideration for return to play decision-making.[47] A prospective study by the National Collegiate Athletic Association Division III women's basketball and soccer players found that a hamstring-to-quadriceps ratio less than 0.6 was associated with noncontact leg injuries.[48,49]

It remains controversial whether bracing should be used on return to sports after operation. The risk of graft injury is significantly higher in young patients, with the greatest risk in those aged 10–19 years.[33] Up to 29.5% of young athletes sustain a second ACL injury within the first 2 years after returning to sports.[31] Wright and Fetzer[50] studied the effect of a functional ACL brace on return to activities following ACL reconstruction. In their series, which consisted primarily of adult patients, bracing had no significant impact on preventing injury.[50] However, as younger athletes also display greater risk-taking behavior, Wright and Fetzer[50] still recommend the use of postoperative ACL braces in children and adolescents.

SUMMARY

The incidence ACL injury in children and adolescents is increasing, as is the number of ACL reconstructions being performed in these young patients. Physeal sparing ACL reconstruction is safe in skeletally immature individuals with ACL tear and may prevent chondral and meniscal injury while allowing them to return to sports and activities. Although the risk of ACL injury in children may be similar in males and females, females are at greater risk of sustaining an ACL tear starting in adolescence. Anatomic, hormonal, biomechanical, and neuromuscular factors seem to contribute to the increased risk of ACL injury among females.

REFERENCES

1. Stanitski C, Harvell JC, F F. Observations on acute knee haemarthrosis in children and adolescents. *J Pediatr Orthop*. 1993;13(4):506–510.
2. Arendt E, Dick R. Knee injury patterns among men and women in collegiate basketball and soccer. NCAA data and review of literature. *Am J Sport Med*. 1995;23(6):694–701.
3. Agel J, Arendt EA, Bershadsky B. Anterior cruciate ligament injury in national collegiate athletic association basketball and soccer: a 13-year review. *Am J Sport Med*. 2005;33(4):524–530. https://doi.org/10.1177/0363546504269937.
4. Lindenfeld TN, Schmitt DJ, Hendy MP, Mangine RE, Noyes F. Incidence of injury in indoor soccer. *Am J Sport Med*. 1994;22(3):364–371.
5. Harmon KG, Ireland M. Gender differences in noncontact anterior cruciate ligament injuries. *Clin Sport Med*. 2000;19(2):287–302.
6. LaBella CR, Hennrikus W, Hewett TE. Anterior cruciate ligament injuries: diagnosis, treatment, and prevention. *Pediatrics*. 2014;133(5):e1437–e1450. https://doi.org/10.1542/peds.2014-0623.
7. Malinzak RA, Colby SM, Kirkendall DT, Yu B, Garrett W. A comparison of knee joint motion patterns between men and women in selected athletic tasks. *Clin Biomech*. 2001;16(5):438–445.
8. Griffin LY, Albohm MJ, Arendt EA, et al. Understanding and preventing noncontact anterior cruciate ligament injuries: a review of the Hunt Valley II meeting, January 2005. *Am J Sport Med*. 2006;34(9):1512–1532. https://doi.org/10.1177/0363546506286866.
9. Stracciolini A, Casciano R, Levey Friedman H, Meehan WP, Micheli LJ. Pediatric sports injuries: an age comparison of children versus adolescents. *Am J Sports Med*. 2013;41(8):1922–1929. https://doi.org/10.1177/0363546513490644.
10. Stracciolini A, Stein CJ, Zurakowski D, Meehan WP, Myer GD, Micheli LJ. Anterior cruciate ligament injuries in pediatric athletes presenting to sports medicine clinic: a comparison of males and females through growth and development. *Sports Health*. 2015;7(2):130–136. https://doi.org/10.1177/1941738114554768.
11. Smith HC, Vacek P, Johnson RJ, et al. Risk factors for anterior cruciate ligament injury: a review of the literature - part 1: neuromuscular and anatomic risk. *Sports Health*. 2012;4(1):69–78. https://doi.org/10.1177/1941738111428281.
12. Smith HC, Vacek P, Johnson RJ, et al. Risk factors for anterior cruciate ligament injury: a review of the literature–part 2: hormonal, genetic, cognitive function, previous injury, and extrinsic risk factors. *Sports Health*. 2012;4(2):155–161. https://doi.org/10.1177/1941738111428282.
13. Dare DM, Fabricant PD, McCarthy MM, et al. Increased lateral tibial slope is a risk factor for pediatric anterior cruciate ligament injury: an MRI-based case-control study of 152 patients. *Am J Sports Med*. 2015;43(7):1632–1639. https://doi.org/10.1177/0363546515579182.
14. Beynnon BD, Hall JS, Sturnick DR, et al. Increased slope of the lateral tibial plateau subchondral bone is associated with greater risk of noncontact ACL injury in females but not in males a prospective cohort study with a nested. *Matched Case Control Anal*. 2014. https://doi.org/10.1177/0363546514523721.
15. Kocher MS, Mandiga R, Klingele K, Bley L, Micheli LJ. Anterior cruciate ligament injury versus tibial spine fracture in the skeletally immature knee. *J Pediatr Orthop*. 2004. https://doi.org/10.1097/01241398-200403000-00010.
16. Everhart JS, Flanigan DC, Simon RA, Chaudhari AMW. Association of noncontact anterior cruciate ligament injury with presence and thickness of a bony ridge on the anteromedial aspect of the femoral intercondylar notch. *Am J Sports Med*. 2010;38(8):1667–1673. https://doi.org/10.1177/0363546510367424.
17. Davis TJ, Shelbourne KD, Klootwyk TE. Correlation of the intercondylar notch width of the femur to the width of the anterior and posterior cruciate ligaments. *Knee Surg Sport Traumatol Arthrosc*. 1999;7(4):209–214. https://doi.org/10.1007/s001670050150.
18. Whitney DC, Sturnick DR, Vacek PM, et al. Relationship between the risk of suffering a first-time noncontact ACL

injury and geometry of the femoral notch and ACL: a prospective cohort study with a nested case-control analysis. *Am J Sports Med.* 2014;42(8):1796–1805. https://doi.org/10.1177/0363546514534182.

19. Hewett TE, Myer GD, Ford KR, et al. Biomechanical measures of neuromuscular control and valgus loading of the knee predict anterior cruciate ligament injury risk in female athletes: a prospective study. *Am J Sport Med.* 2005;33(4):492–501. https://doi.org/10.1177/0363546504269591.

20. Hewett TE, Torg JS, Boden B. Video analysis of trunk and knee motion during non-contact anterior cruciate ligament injury in female athletes: lateral trunk and knee abduction motion are combined components of the injury mechanism. *Br J Sport Med.* 2009;43(6):417–422. https://doi.org/10.1136/bjsm.2009.059162.

21. Zazulak BT, Hewett TE, Reeves NP, Goldberg B, Cholewicki J. Deficits in neuromuscular control of the trunk predict knee injury risk: a prospective biomechanical-epidemiologic study. *Am J Sports Med.* 2007;35(7):1123–1130. https://doi.org/10.1177/0363546507301585.

22. Khayambashi K, Ghoddosi N, Straub RK, Powers C. Hip muscle strength Predicts noncontact anterior cruciate ligament injury in male and female athletes: a prospective study. Epub 2015 Dec 8 *Am J Sport Med.* 2016;44(2):355–361. https://doi.org/10.1177/0363546515616237.

23. Khayambashi K, Ghoddosi N, Straub RK, Powers CM. Hip muscle strength predicts noncontact anterior cruciate ligament injury in male and female athletes: a prospective study. *Am J Sports Med.* 2015:1–7. https://doi.org/10.1177/0363546515616237.

24. Kocher MS, Micheli LJ, Zurakowski D, Luke A. Partial tears of the anterior cruciate ligament in children and adolescents. *Am J Sport Med.* 2002;30(5):697–703.

25. Graf BK, Lange RH, Fujisaki CK, Landry GL, Saluja R. Anterior cruciate ligament tears in skeletally immature patients: meniscal pathology at presentation and after attempted conservative treatment. *Arthroscopy.* 1992;8(2):229–233.

26. McCarroll JR, Shelbourne KD, Patel D. Anterior cruciate ligament injuries in young athletes. Recommendations for treatment and rehabilitation. *Sport Med.* 1995;20(2):117–127.

27. Janarv PM, Nyström A, Werner S, Hirsch G. Anterior cruciate ligament injuries in skeletally immature patients. *J Pediatr Orthop.* 1996;16(5):673–677.

28. Pressman AE, Letts RM, Jarvis J. Anterior cruciate ligament tears in children: an analysis of operative versus nonoperative treatment. *J Pediatr Orthop.* 1997;17(4):505–511.

29. Aichroth PM, Patel DV, Zorrilla P. The natural history and treatment of rupture of the anterior cruciate ligament in children and adolescents. A prospective review. *J Bone Jt Surg Br.* 2002;84(1):38–41.

30. Finlayson CJ, Nasreddine A, Kocher MS. Current concepts of diagnosis and management of ACL injuries in skeletally immature athletes. *Phys Sportsmed.* 2010. https://doi.org/10.3810/psm.2010.06.1789.

31. Dekker TJ, Rush JK, Schmitz MR. What's new in pediatric and adolescent anterior cruciate ligament injuries?

32. Greulich WW, Pyle S. *Radiographic Atlas of Skeletal Development of the Hand and Wrist.* 2nd ed. Stanford, CA: Stanford University Press; 1959.

33. Kaeding CC, Aros B, Pedroza A, et al. Allograft versus autograft anterior cruciate ligament reconstruction: predictors of failure from a MOON prospective longitudinal cohort. *Sports Health.* 2011;3(1):73–81. https://doi.org/10.1177/1941738110386185.

34. Micheli LJ, Rask B, Gerberg L. Anterior cruciate ligament reconstruction in patients who are prepubescent. *Clin Orthop Relat Res.* 1999;364:40–47.

35. Kocher MS, Garg S, Micheli L. Physeal sparing reconstruction of the anterior cruciate ligament in skeletally immature prepubescent children and adolescents. *J Bone Jt Surg Am.* 2005;87(11):2371–2379. https://doi.org/10.2106/JBJS.D.02802.

36. Anderson AF. Transepiphyseal replacement of the anterior cruciate ligament in skeletally immature patients: a preliminary report. *J Bone Jt Surg Am.* 2003;85(7):1255–1263.

37. Pierce TP, Issa K, Festa A, Scillia AJ, McInerney VK. Pediatric anterior cruciate ligament reconstruction a systematic review of transphyseal versus physeal-sparing techniques. *Am J Sport Med.* 2016. https://doi.org/10.1177/0363546516638079 Clinical.

38. Cruz AI, Fabricant PD, McGraw M, Rozell JC, Ganley TJ, Wells L. All-epiphyseal ACL reconstruction in children: review of safety and early complications. *J Pediatr Orthop.* 2015;0(0):1–6. https://doi.org/10.1097/BPO.0000000000000606.

39. Stadelmaier DM, Arnoczky SP, Dodds J, Ross H. The effect of drilling and soft tissue grafting across open growth plates. A histologic study. *Am J Sport Med.* 1995;23(4):431–435.

40. Calvo R, Figueroa D, Gili F, et al. Transphyseal anterior cruciate ligament reconstruction in patients with open physes: 10-year follow-up study. *Am J Sports Med.* 2015;43(2):289–294. https://doi.org/10.1177/0363546514557939.

41. Hui C, Roe J, Ferguson D, Waller A, Salmon L, Pinczewski L. Outcome of anatomic transphyseal anterior cruciate ligament reconstruction in Tanner stage 1 and 2 patients with open physes. *Am J Sport Med.* 2012;40(5):1093–1098. https://doi.org/10.1177/0363546512438508.

42. Reid D, Leigh W, Wilkins S, Willis R, Twaddle BWS. A 10-year retrospective review of functional outcomes of adolescent anterior cruciate ligament reconstruction. *J Pediatr Orthop.* 2017. https://doi.org/10.1097/BPO.0000000000000594.

43. Kushner AM, Adam M, Kiefer AW, et al. Training the developing brain Part II: cognitive considerations for youth instruction and feedback. *Curr Sport Med Rep.* 2015;14(3):235–243. https://doi.org/10.1002/aur.1474. Replication.

44. van Melick N, van Cingel REH, Brooijmans F, et al. Evidence-based clinical practice update: practice guidelines for anterior cruciate ligament rehabilitation based on a systematic review and multidisciplinary consensus. *Br J Sports Med.* 2016:bjsports-2015–095898. https://doi.org/10.1136/bjsports-2015-095898.

45. Wilk KE, Arrigo C. Rehabilitation principles of the anterior cruciate ligament reconstructed knee: twelve steps for successful progression and return to play. *Clin Sport Med.* 2017;36(1):189–232. https://doi.org/10.1016/j.csm.2016.08.012.

46. Chicorelli AM, Micheli LJ, Kelly M, Zurakowski D, Macdougall R. Return to sport after anterior cruciate ligament reconstruction in the skeletally immature athlete. *Clin J Sport Med.* 2016;26:266–271.

47. Kyritsis P, Bahr R, Landreau P, Miladi R, Witvrouw E. Likelihood of ACL graft rupture: not meeting six clinical discharge criteria before return to sport is associated with a four times greater risk of rupture. *Br J Sports Med.* 2016;50(15):946–951. https://doi.org/10.1136/bjsports-2015-095908.

48. Kim D, Hong J. Hamstring to quadriceps strength ratio and noncontact leg injuries: a prospective study during one season. *Isokinet Exerc Sci.* 2011;19(1):1–6. https://doi.org/0.3233/IES-2011-0406.

49. Myer GD, Ford KR, Barber Foss KD, Liu C, Nick TG, Hewett T. The relationship of hamstrings and quadriceps strength to anterior cruciate ligament injury in female athletes. *Clin J Sport Med.* 2009;19(1):3–8. https://doi.org/10.1097/JSM.0b013e318190bddb.

50. Wright RW, Fetzer G. Bracing after ACL reconstruction: a systematic review. *Clin Orthop Relat Res.* 2007;455:162–168. https://doi.org/10.1097/BLO.0b013e31802c9360.

CHAPTER 8

Special Considerations: Revision Anterior Cruciate Ligament

MICHELLE E. KEW, MD • KIERAN R. BHATTACHARYA, BCH • MARK D. MILLER, MD

INTRODUCTION

Although the majority of patients who undergo anterior cruciate ligament (ACL) reconstruction (ACLR) have favorable short-term results, there is still a chance for a reinjury or failure. A systematic review of studies found that the ACL graft rupture rate at 5 years or more ranged from 1.8% to 10.4%, with a pooled percentage of 5.8%.[1] In one study, young female soccer players who returned to play after ACLRs had a graft tear rate of 15% during a 5-year follow-up period.[2]

The causes of failed ACLR are variable and multifactorial; therefore, a comprehensive history taking, physical examination, and radiographic imaging should be performed for planning and completing a successful revision.

CAUSES OF GRAFT FAILURE

Identifying the cause of ACL failure is imperative to a successful revision surgery. The leading causes of ACL graft rupture have been found to be technical errors and recurrent trauma. The Multicenter ACL Revision Study (MARS) group reported that surgeons performing revision ACLR attributed graft failure to trauma (32%), technical error (24%), biologic factors (7%), or a combination of these factors (37%)[3] (Fig. 8.1), with a follow-up study confirming the multifactorial cause of graft rupture.[4] In cases where there is no significant traumatic episode or obvious technical problems with the previous ACLR procedure, the cause of failure is defined as biologic likely owing to the failure of graft incorporation.

The first and most common technical error was found to be femoral tunnel malposition (80%), followed by tibial tunnel malposition (37%).[3] Correct positioning of bone tunnels avoids nonphysiologic strain patterns of the graft throughout the functional range and reduces the chance of graft failure or limitation in knee motion.[5] When evaluating the anteroposterior stability of the knee after ACLR, it was found that an increase in postoperative knee laxity was most likely due to malposition of the bone tunnels.[6] An anteriorly placed femoral tunnel causes loss of knee flexion because of the

excessive graft tension during flexion, whereas a posteriorly placed femoral tunnel causes laxity in flexion, along with increased graft tension, during full extension of the knee.[7,8] Initially the ACLR techniques involved placing the graft close to the central axis of the tibia and femur, and although this placement restores anteroposterior stability, it is inadequate for resisting rotational loads.[9] Furthermore, anterior positioning of the femoral and tibial tunnels was associated with tunnel enlargement. It has been shown that patients with an enlarged femoral tunnel have significantly smaller femoral angles than those of patients with an unenlarged femoral tunnel.[10] The exact mechanism of femoral tunnel enlargement is unknown, but it has been characterized as having four different shapes: cavitary, mushroom, conical, and linear as the most common[11] (Fig. 8.2). We have found that tibial tunnel widening is often greater than that on the femoral side, but we are unaware of any descriptive features. No clinical consequences have been associated with tunnel enlargement,[10–12] but tunnel enlargement can make revision ACLR more challenging and may require a two-stage approach.

The second technical consideration is appropriate hardware placement and the need to monitor for subsequent hardware failure. Fixation is critical to a stable ACL graft and prevents graft movement in the tunnels. Kurosaka et al. noted that graft fixation is weakest in the immediate postoperative period; therefore, hardware must be appropriately placed to ensure adequate graft tensioning and placement. Interference screws should be placed with <30 degrees divergence in the femoral tunnel and with <15 degrees divergence in the tibial tunnel in order to appropriately secure the graft.[13] Placement of interference screws must be meticulous to ensure placement outside the bone tunnel without damage to the graft itself (Fig. 8.3), as well as to confirm placement with a bony interface (Fig. 8.4).[14] Hamstring graft hardware failure can occur due to either poor positioning of the endoscopic fastener or lack of adequate cortical contact.[15]

Bony malalignment can also lead to ACL graft rupture. Varus malalignment and increased tibial slope have both been found to affect ACLR by increasing the stress on the ACL graft.[16] Studies have shown that increased tibial slope leads to a more anteriorly translated tibia,[17] and as the ACL is the primary restraint to this motion,[18] it will see an increased stress. A meta-analysis noted that increased tibial slope, specifically the lateral tibial posterior slope, is associated with increased risk of ACL injury,[19] and Christensen et al.[20] furthered this notion and noted that increased lateral

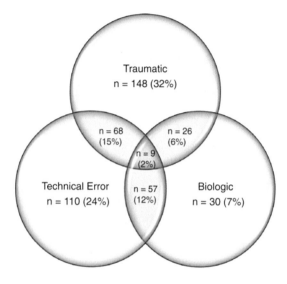

FIG. 8.1 Leading causes of anterior cruciate ligament graft rupture. Reproduced from Wright RW, Huston LJ, Spindler KP, et al. Descriptive epidemiology of the multicenter ACL revision study (MARS) cohort. *Am J Sports Med*. October 2010;38(10):1979–1986.

tibial slope increases the risks of early ACL graft tear. A longitudinal study with 20-year follow-up noted that a posterior tibial slope greater than 12 degrees was the strongest predictor of repeat ACL injury. This data suggests that critical evaluation by imaging techniques should be performed preoperatively, including measurement of tibial slope, in addition to the other radiographic parameters discussed. Studies have evaluated the use of anterior closing wedge tibial osteotomy prior to a revision ACL procedure to correct increased posterior tibial slope. A cadaveric study demonstrated that a 10-degree anterior tibial osteotomy resulted in decreased anterior tibial translation and ACL force, with a 200-N tibiofemoral compression force.[21] This technique has been validated in vivo (Fig. 8.5) and found to restore knee stability and to allow return to play at a similar level before operation.[21]

Traumatic rupture of an ACL graft can be due to an acute event or repetitive microtrauma that slowly weakens the graft. Physical therapy regimens that emphasize aggressive and early postoperative motion can also lead to traumatic failure of primary ACLR.[22] This can be attributed to the relative weakness of the ACL graft during the first postoperative year, as grafts have been shown to have 30% strength and 50% resistance of the native ACL at evaluation after 1 year.[23] Multiple microtraumautic episodes can also cause chronic loosening of the graft and ultimately lead to failure. These episodes occur during high-level athletic activities involving jumping and cutting movements.[24,25]

Failure to recognize limb malalignment or injury to the posteromedial or posterolateral corner (PLC) can indirectly lead to ACL graft failure. Corner injuries are rarely isolated but occur in conjunction with ACL and/or posterior cruciate ligament (PCL) injuries.[26] These injuries augment the force sustained by the graft and

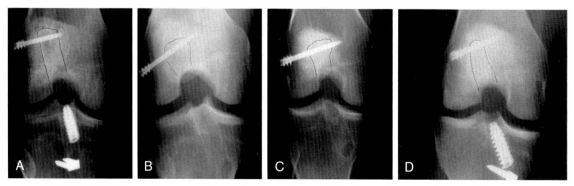

FIG. 8.2 **(A–D)** The most common shapes for femoral tunnel widening are linear, cavitary, mushroom, and conical. Reproduced from Klein JP, Linter DM, Downs D, Vavrenka K. The incidence and significant of femoral tunnel widening after quadrupled hamstring anterior cruciate ligament reconstruction using femoral cross pin fixation. Arthroscopy. May-June 2003;19(5):470-476.

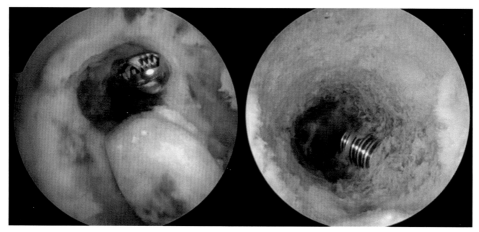

FIG. 8.3 Arthroscopic images showing interference screw in bone tunnel.

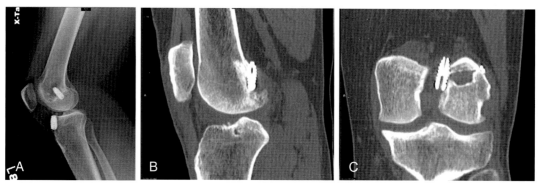

FIG. 8.4 **(A)** Radiographic and **(B** and **C)** computed tomographic images showing interference screw with no cortical contact.

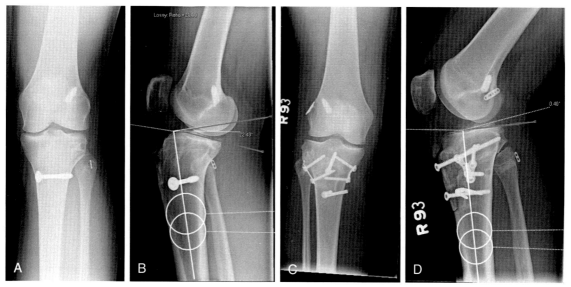

FIG. 8.5 **(A** and **B)** Preoperative and **(C** and **D)** postoperative **(C** and **D)** radiographs of a patient with posterior tibial slope.

lead to an increase in graft attenuation, which leads to graft failure. Another pathologic condition that can contribute to ACL graft tear is varus malalignment of the knee. This can be due to a normal anatomic variant or can be augmented by medial compartment narrowing as a result of prior meniscectomy. Malalignment causes a varus thrust gait and increases the stretching force of the graft.[27] In this case, a valgus high tibial osteotomy can be combined with ACLR for favorable outcomes in returning to sports.[28-30] In cases of chronic ACL-medial collateral ligament (MCL) lesions, it has been suggested that nonoperative management of the MCL injury may lead to chronic valgus instability and rotatory instability, so graft reconstruction in both the ACL and MCL is sometimes recommended[31,32] (Fig. 8.6).

In addition to technical errors and concomitant ligament injuries, graft selection is an important factor in the cause of graft failure. When compared with allografts, autografts used in ACLR were found to be significantly less likely to result in a revision.[33] Another study found that the use of autograft in revisions resulted in patients being 2.78 times less likely to sustain a subsequent graft rupture than those with allografts.[34] The use of freeze-dried, ethylene oxide–sterilized, bone-patellar tendon-bone (BPTB) allografts is also not recommended for ACLR because of the high rates of dissolution of the graft, formation of large femoral cysts, and immune-mediated responses.[35,36] However, reconstructions with nonirradiated, non–chemically treated allografts and allograft-autograft hybrids produced failure rates comparable to those of reconstructions with autografts, but irradiated allograft-autograft hybrids became structurally compromised at higher rates than matched

autograft hamstring controls.[37-39] With respect to autografts, both BPTB and hamstring tendons are popular, but both have specific associated complications. Patellar tendon grafts can cause pain during kneeling or squatting and patellar fractures have been reported after acute trauma.[40] Harvest of the semitendinosus and/or the gracilis tendons for autografts has been demonstrated to result in regeneration of the tendons in 1 year but with reduced cross-sectional area and without any differences between pre- and postoperative isokinetic extension and flexion strength.[41] Furthermore, there is no measurable drawback or benefit from harvesting the semitendinosus-gracilis tendons from the unaffected limb.[42] ACLR is less commonly performed using a patellar tendon autograft from the contralateral knee because of concerns for donor site morbidity, but patients can still achieve symmetry in strength after surgery without donor site pain.[43,44] Alternatively, a graft can be obtained from a quadriceps tendon harvest with or without a bone block and can produce desirable results.[45]

HISTORY

A detailed patient history is important and should include symptoms and mechanism of injury, assessment of function following initial reconstruction, rehabilitation strategy, and description of reinjury. One should discriminate between symptoms of pain or stiffness and true instability and have the patient describe what activities result in a feeling of instability. It is often helpful to ask the patients if they "trust" their knee. Identifying concomitant injuries such as meniscal deficiency, chondral damage, malalignment,

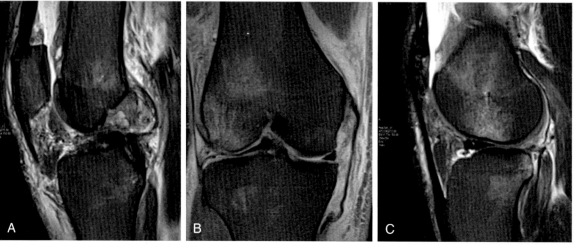

FIG. 8.6 **(A–C)** T2-weighted MRI images showing combined anterior cruciate ligament/medial collateral ligament injury.

or other ligamentous injuries is imperative. The timing of the primary ACLR failure can help predict the cause: early failures (<3 months) are associated with loss of fixation and infection; midterm failures (3–12 months) commonly occur with aggressive physical therapy, unnoticed concomitant ligament injuries, and errors in surgical technique; and late failures (>12 months) are often related to repeat trauma.[46] Operative notes, arthroscopic images, and implant records can be used to plan for hardware removal if necessary. It is also useful to note whether the original femoral tunnel was drilled transtibially or by an independent technique and if the primary reconstruction was double or single bundle.

PHYSICAL EXAMINATION

During the physical examination, it is critical to examine both the affected and unaffected knees to obtain baseline measurements for the patient. In the affected knee, one should examine previous skin incisions, swelling, muscle tone, and range of motion in both the prone and supine positions. The Lachman test should be employed to determine the anterior tibial translation and laxity in comparison to the unaffected contralateral knee, but the test has limited reliability and is more useful for predicting if a patient does not have an ACL injury than for predicting if the ACL is injured.[47] The pivot shift test can also be used with the patient completely relaxed and testing the ACL rotational

stability by mimicking the act of giving way. Posterolateral instability can be diagnosed with the dial test, and although a positive result is usually used to differentiate between an isolated PCL injury and a combination of PLC/PCL injury, it should still not rule out an isolated ACL injury.[48] Anteromedial rotatory instability of the knee can be measured by the Slocum test, and PCL deficiency can be assessed with the posterior draw test and sag sign.[49] Additionally, one can utilize the KT-1000 arthrometer (Medmetric) for more sensitive and reliable measurements of the anterior translation and laxity of the knee.[50,51] An ACL graft rupture can be validly represented by a difference of >3 mm in the anteroposterior knee laxity when compared with a healthy knee or a >10 mm absolute displacement as measured through KT-1000 with a 99% sensitivity.[14] Finally, abnormal or asymmetric gait behaviors, as well as standing limb alignment, should be analyzed, as they can be an indicator of the cause of graft failure.[52]

IMAGING

Although MRI is the "gold standard" for detecting primary ACL tears, it is often insufficient when used alone in the assessment of ACLR failures.[53] The size and location of previous tunnels are estimated using bilateral standing radiographs and a true lateral radiograph (Fig. 8.7). Plain radiographs can be used to assess hardware type, tunnel osteolysis, and patellofemoral pathology.

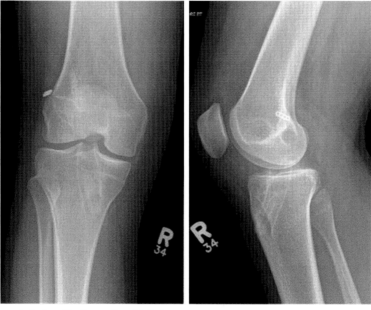

FIG. 8.7 Radiographs of failed anterior cruciate ligament reconstruction.

Weight-bearing posteroanterior and/or anteroposterior views are important in evaluating joint space and joint space narrowing if degenerative changes are suspected. Furthermore, in cases of degeneration and posterolateral or posteromedial laxity, long-standing films are necessary to assess alignment. Varus stress radiography can be used to identify PLC injuries by providing information about the resulting pathologic laxity.[54] MRI is more useful than plain radiographs in depicting the position of preexisting tunnels as well as the status of the graft. MRI can also be employed to evaluate meniscal and cartilage lesions. However, MRI has limitations, as it cannot be used to determine the functionality of the graft and the signal can be disrupted by metal implants or edema around implants. Ultimately, computed tomography (CT) with or without 3D reconstruction is the superior imaging modality (Fig. 8.8) for exact characterization of bone tunnels when compared with radiography or MRI.[55,56]

ONE-STAGE VERSUS TWO-STAGE REVISIONS

There are a variety of ways to perform a revision ACLR, and it should be first determined whether the ACL can be repaired in one operation or if the process needs several stages. The most common indications for a two-stage revision are enlarged bone tunnels from osteolysis and malpositioned preexisting tunnels that interfere with new revision reconstruction tunnel placement.[57] Femoral tunnel lysis of ≥15 mm and tibial tunnel lysis of ≥15 mm in any plane on a CT scan are considered absolute indications for two-stage revisions, as these misplaced or enlarged bone tunnels must be filled with cancellous bone.[58,59] Other deciding factors between a single- and two-stage revisions include presence of active infection, loss of extension >5 degrees, and loss of flexion >20 degrees.[57,59–61] The primary disadvantage of a two-stage revision is the necessary 3- to 6-month delay for healing of the cancellous bone.[59] Apart from the associated risks of two surgeries and two exposures to anesthesia, the period of knee instability with a two-stage revision can be detrimental to female athletes or those with physically demanding occupations. Only 8%–9% of revision ACLR procedures require two stages.[3]

PROCEDURE
Preoperative
Osteolysis of the bone tunnels should be characterized with CT scan using multiple orthogonal views. Tunnel osteolysis of ≥15 mm diameter in any plane of space

is a general indication for a two-stage procedure. Also, if the previous tunnel would compromise the revision tunnel a two-stage procedure should be considered. Furthermore, sagittal CT cuts should be taken to measure the tibial tunnel angle, which can be used as a reference point for tibial guidewire placement.

Setup
As with the primary ACLR the revision procedure is performed with the patient positioned supine on the operating table. After inducing anesthesia, both the nonoperative and operative legs are examined using the Lachman, pivot shift, anterior drawer, and range of motion tests. Careful note should be taken of the posterolateral, valgus, and varus instability.

Hardware Removal
Arthroscopic images and implant records can be used to assess if hardware removal is necessary. Implant removal can be difficult and time-consuming and could create further bony defects, so implants should only be removed if they interfere with revision tunnel placement. Metallic hardware should be removed if a two-stage procedure is necessary due to tunnel widening for anatomic and overlapping tunnels.[46] Regardless of whether a surgeon plans to remove hardware, he or she should gain access to operative reports of the primary reconstruction to understand how the hardware was placed and to ensure that the proper tools are available.

Bone Grafting in Two-Stage Procedures
In cases in which the degree of osteolysis requires bone grafting as the first stage procedure, it is necessary to debride all soft tissue and remnant graft out of the tunnel. Options for bone grafts include allograft bone dowels, allograft chips, allograft femoral head, commercially available bone substitutes, and autogenous bone graft from the iliac crest.[46] One review of autogenous bone grafting of tibial tunnels found significantly higher occupying ratio, union ratio, and bone mineral density after 24 weeks than those after 12 weeks, and this suggests that this increase in time provides a more favorable environment for ACL graft revision.[62] Bone dowels have been shown to be an alternative to cancellous bone grafting.[63] This method of allografting can be chosen at precise diameters, stacked to equal adequate tunnel length and inserted by arthroscopic assistance.[46] The healing of any cancellous bone grafting takes 3–6 months and should be assessed by CT scan within that period to ensure adequate incorporation.

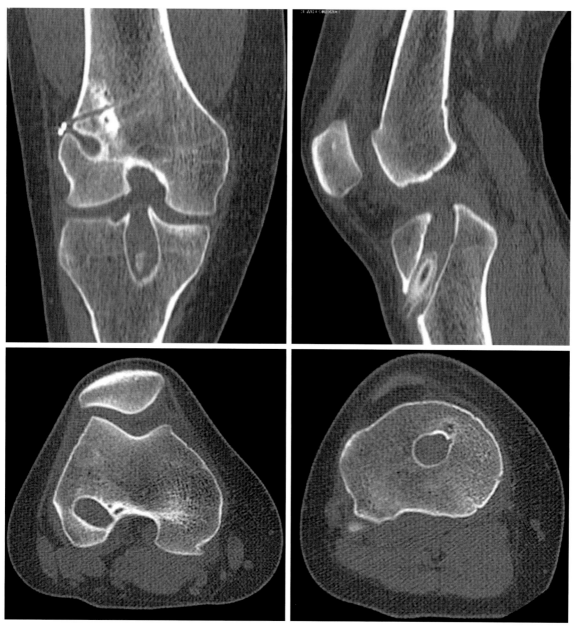

FIG. 8.8 Computed tomographic scans of failed anterior cruciate ligament reconstruction showing bone tunnels.

Graft Fixation

In revision ACLR the weakest components are the fixation sites and may cause biomechanical failure.[64,65] The general consensus is that the normal ACL will undergo forces of up to 500 N during daily activities; therefore, a graft fixation construct should be able to withstand at least that force.[66] In femoral and/or tibial tunnels with gross osteolysis or gross convergence, extracortical fixation can be achieved with larger-diameter interference screws. This fixation method has been found to be beneficial in tendon-to-bone incorporation by allowing for direct contact healing and preventing formation of a fibrous layer.[67] Additionally, one study demonstrated decreased surgical failures with femoral fixation at the joint line with interference screws compared with nonaperture fixations.[68] In deciding what type of interference screws are appropriate, one should note that there is a concern that metal femoral screws might tear the soft tissue graft, leading to early failure.[69] However, in one study that examined 790 knees, there was found to be no significant difference between bioabsorbable and metallic interference screws, except that a knee joint effusion was more common among bioabsorbable screws.[70] Stacked screws should not be employed in single-stage revisions, as they may compromise graft fixation and increase risk of failure.[65] Furthermore, screw divergence from the tunnel should not exceed 15 degrees.[64] Good fixation is paramount, and therefore, interference screws need to interfere, cortical buttons need to engage the cortex, and interosseous fixation with backup suture should always be considered with revision ACL procedures.

CASE EXAMPLE: TWO-STAGE PROCEDURE

A 51-year-old male who had an ACLR before 1 year presented with left-knee pain. He reported doing well for about 1 year until falling and experiencing a "pop" and subsequent "cracking" in his left knee. He presented with recurrent left-knee pain, instability, and swelling. He stated that he did not "trust" his knee. Prolonged walking and lateral movements aggravated symptoms, and he denied relief in symptoms from activity modification, RICE (rest, ice, compression, elevation), using brace wear, and home exercise program. A CT scan showed changes of an ACLR with minimal osseous material surrounding a tibial interference screw that extended 1.1 cm from the anterior tibial cortex as well as osseous formation around the femoral screw with cystic changes around the femoral tunnel (Fig. 8.9). Femoral tunnels and tibial tunnels were measured at 13 and 16 mm, respectively.

A two-stage procedure was decided upon due to the widening of bone tunnels. The first stage of revision ACLR consisted of femoral and tibial bone dowel allografts, along with arthroscopic partial medial and lateral meniscectomies. The small lateral meniscal tear was debrided. The femoral and tibial sides of the prior ACL graft were debrided completely, and a curette was used to sound the femoral tunnel in hyperflexion. The prior interference screws and sheaths were removed without complication. Partially threaded drills were used to drill to 12 mm through the femoral tunnel (Fig. 8.10), and a flexible reamer was used to drill to 14 mm. After using

a scope to confirm that there were good bony edges on all aspects of the tunnel, a 14-mm × 26-mm bone dowel was used to graft the tunnel (Fig. 8.11).

On the tibial side, the prominent tibial interference screw was removed without issue. The tunnel was then serially reamed up to 16 mm, and a scope was again used to confirm that there were good bony edges throughout the tunnel (Fig. 8.12). After a shaver was used to debride all the remaining graft and suture, a 16-mm × 26-mm allograft dowel was placed (Fig. 8.13), with an arthroscope used to confirm it was not advanced too far. There was about 10 mm of space remaining distally in the tunnel, so 5 cc of cancellous allograft chips were packed in finger-tight.

Two weeks after the operation, the patient was found to have excellent knee stability and appropriate range of motion.

The patient returned to the clinic 4 months later for a scheduled stage 2 ACLR revision preoperative evaluation. Through CT scans, his previously inserted bone dowels were found to be well-integrated into the bone tunnels (Fig. 8.14), and it was thus decided to proceed with the scheduled second surgery.

CASE EXAMPLE: SINGLE-STAGE PROCEDURE

A 21-year-old male presented with right-knee pain. He was status post right ACLR nearly 1 year prior and sustained a noncontact twisting injury while playing soccer 3 weeks prior to presenting with immediate pain and effusion. Presenting symptoms included right-knee instability and recurrent swelling, with pain aggravated by lateral movements, pivoting, twisting, jumping, and athletic activity. MRI showed tearing of the ACL graft with associated medial meniscal tear and CT showed a reusable tibial tunnel and a previous femoral tunnel that would not overlap with the proposed femoral tunnel (Fig. 8.15). Furthermore, there was no significant osteolysis surrounding the tunnels. It was determined that a one-stage revision was appropriate with the use of a BPTB graft and simultaneous bone grafting of the prior femoral tunnel along with medial meniscus repair through a meniscectomy.

During the revision procedure, the patellar tendon graft and bone plugs were harvested and they measured 50 mm × 12 mm. The prior hardware and sutures were removed from the proximal tibia. The ACL and tibial footprints were then debrided with a large shaver. The femoral tunnel was identified, with its center easily visible because of the intact remnants of the previous graft. A guidewire for the ACL was

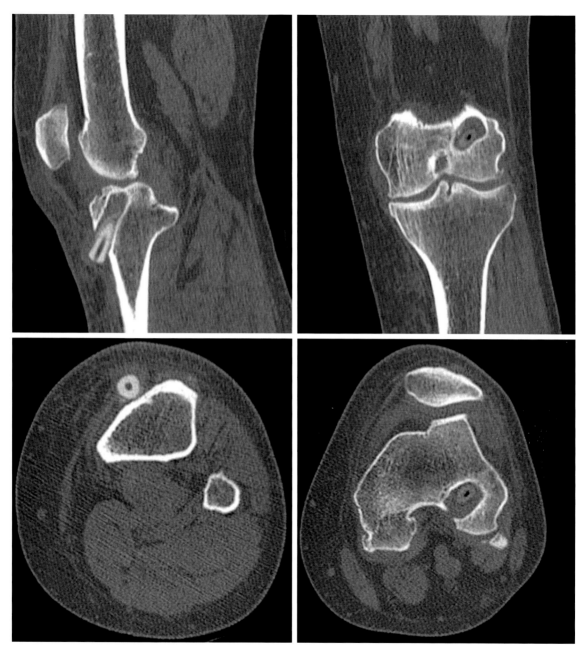

FIG. 8.9 A computed tomographic scan showing minimal osseous material surrounding a tibial interference screw and little osseous formation around the femoral screw.

placed in the femoral tunnel and was passed through the lateral side of the leg. Then, from the previous tibial tunnel, the ACL guide was used to recreate a 55-degree tunnel with a guidewire and then reamer was used to create the new tibial tunnel. All remnants of the previous ACL graft were debrided from the femoral tunnel. A Cloward Dowel #12 was delivered through the tibial tunnel without difficulty and placed in the femoral tunnel, and a burr was used to debride the edges of the plug.

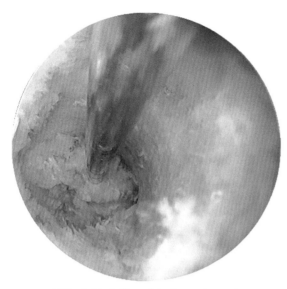

FIG. 8.10 Drilling of the femoral tunnel.

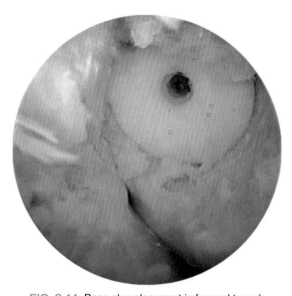

FIG. 8.11 Bone plug placement in femoral tunnel.

The cortex for the ACL was drilled 25 mm deep with a sled to protect the femoral condyle and a reamer was used to ream to 25 mm for the femoral tunnel. An interference screw was used on the femoral side with excellent fixation strength, and a Stryker ACL interference screw was used on the tibial side. Finally, 20 cc of cancellous chips were used to graft the patellar and tibial defects created from harvesting the patellar tendon.

POSTOPERATIVE REHABILITATION

These is no standard postoperative course for patients who have undergone revision ACLR; the variability depends on factors such as age, athletic expectations, graft type, and mechanism of primary ACLR failure. However, initial emphasis is placed on restoring quadriceps activation, restoring tibiofemoral and patellofemoral range of motion, and managing joint effusion.[57] Ankle pumps, heel slides, and straight leg raises can be started immediately after operation to help maximize quadriceps strength.[64,71] Moreover, knee braces can be used to stabilize the knee until quadriceps have returned to adequate strength and can allow for earlier involvement in weight-bearing exercises.[71] Full range of motion should be achieved by 6 weeks, whereas running and other aggressive aerobic activities should be delayed for a minimum of 6 months, and finally, an athlete should not return to competitive play before 9–12 months.[64,65,71]

RESULTS

Athletes who underwent revision ACLRs returned to their usual sport significantly less often within 1 year and demonstrated declined Marx activity scores at 2-year follow-up when compared with matched groups undergoing primary ACLRs.[72,73] The rerupture rate of revision procedures was found to be three to four times higher than that of primary reconstructions in a meta-analysis using a minimum of 2 years of follow-up.[74] Moreover, patients who underwent a third or higher revision were 25.8 times more likely to experience a graft rerupture and 4.7 times more likely to go through additional procedures within 2 years of the third or higher revision surgery.[74] Some independent risk factors for subsequent surgery within 2 years on the ipsilateral knee after a revision procedure include age <20 years and the use of allograft tissue for the revision.[75]

FUTURE CONSIDERATIONS

One promising new method to circumvent the 3–6 month spacing of the two-stage revision in the presence of gross osteolysis is to fill the bone void with calcium phosphate cement and drill a new tunnel right through the construct. However, this method is currently in the experimental stage and the only results produced have been in cadaveric studies.[76,77] Revision ACL is an area of express interest, and new techniques and options are currently in testing and may be developed in the future.

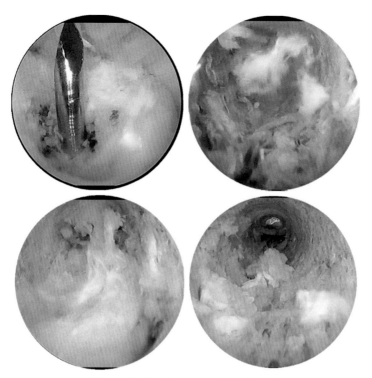

FIG. 8.12 Serial reaming of tibial tunnel.

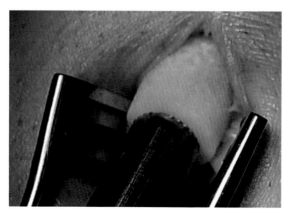

FIG. 8.13 Placement of tibial bone plug.

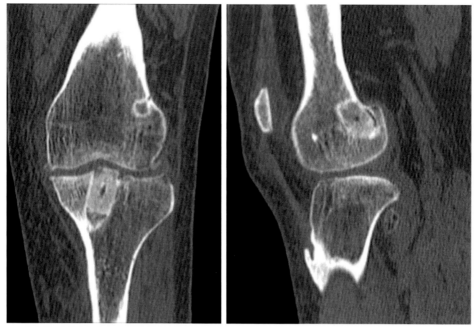

FIG. 8.14 CT scan showing partial integration of femoral and complete integration of tibial bone dowels into respective bone tunnels.

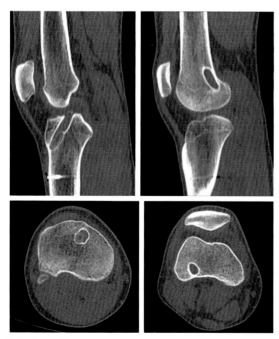

FIG. 8.15 CT scan showing reusable tibial tunnel and previous femoral tunnel that would not overlap with proposed femoral tunnel.

REFERENCES

1. Wright RW, Magnussen RA, Dunn WR, Spindler KP. Ipsilateral graft and contralateral ACL rupture at five years or more following ACL reconstruction: a systematic review. *J Bone Jt Surg Ser A.* 2011;93(12):1159–1165. https://doi.org/10.2106/JBJS.J.00898.
2. Allen MM, Pareek A, Krych AJ, et al. Are female soccer players at an increased risk of second anterior cruciate ligament injury compared with their athletic peers? *Am J Sports Med.* 2016;44(10):2492–2498. https://doi.org/10.1177/0363546516648439.
3. Wright RW, Huston LJ, Spindler KP, et al. Descriptive epidemiology of the multicenter ACL revision study (MARS) cohort. *Am J Sports Med.* 2010;38(10):1979–1986. https://doi.org/10.1177/0363546510378645.
4. Chen JL, Allen CR, Stephens TE, et al. Differences in mechanisms of failure, intraoperative findings, and surgical characteristics between single- and multiple-revision ACL reconstructions: a MARS cohort study. *Am J Sports Med.* 2013;41(7):1571–1578. https://doi.org/10.1177/0363546513487980.
5. Dargel J, Gotter M, Mader K, Pennig D, Koebke J, Schmidt-Wiethoff R. Biomechanics of the anterior cruciate ligament and implications for surgical reconstruction. *Strateg Trauma Limb Reconstr.* 2007;2(1):1–12. https://doi.org/10.1007/s11751-007-0016-6.

6. Rupp S, Müller B, Seil R. Knee laxity after ACL reconstruction with a BPTB graft. *Knee Surg Sport Traumatol Arthrosc.* 2001;9(2):72–76. https://doi.org/10.1007/s001670000177.

7. Carson EW, Anisko EM, Restrepo C. Revision anterior cruciate ligament reconstruction: etiology of failures and clinical results. *J Knee Surg.* 2004;17(3):127–132.

8. Kamath GV, Redfern JC, Greis PE, Burks RT. Revision anterior cruciate ligament reconstruction. *Am J Sports Med.* 2011;39(1):199–217. https://doi.org/10.1177/0363546510370929.

9. Woo SL, Kanamori A, Zeminski J, Yagi M, Papageorgiou CFF. The effectiveness of reconstruction of the anterior cruciate ligament with hamstrings and patellar tendon. A cadaveric study comparing anterior tibial and rotational loads. *J Bone Jt Surg.* 2002;84-A(6):907–914.

10. Segawa H, Omori G, Tomita S, Koga Y. Bone tunnel enlargement after anterior cruciate ligament reconstruction using hamstring tendons. *Knee Surg Sport Traumatol Arthrosc.* 2001;9(4):206–210. https://doi.org/10.1007/s001670100201.

11. Klein JP, Lintner DM, Downs D, Vavrenka K. The incidence and significance of femoral tunnel widening after quadrupled hamstring anterior cruciate ligament reconstruction using femoral cross pin fixation. *Arthrosc J Arthrosc Relat Surg.* 2003;19(5):470–476. https://doi.org/10.1053/jars.2003.50106.

12. Xu Y, Ao Y, Wang J, Yu J, Cui G. Relation of tunnel enlargement and tunnel placement after single-bundle anterior cruciate ligament reconstruction. *Arthrosc J Arthrosc Relat Surg.* 2011;27(7):923–932. https://doi.org/10.1016/j.arthro.2011.02.020.

13. Dworsky BD, Jewell BF, Bach BR. Interference screw divergence in endoscopic anterior cruciate ligament reconstruction. *Arthroscopy.* 1996;12(1):45–49. https://doi.org/10.1016/S0749-8063(96)90218-2.

14. Samitier G, Marcano AI, Alentorn-Geli E, Cugat R, Farmer KW, Moser MW. Failure of anterior cruciate ligament reconstruction. *Arch Bone Jt Surg.* 2015;3(4):220–240. https://doi.org/10.1016/j.csm.2012.08.015.

15. Getelman MH, Friedman MJ. Revision anterior cruciate ligament reconstruction surgery. *J Am Acad Orthop Surg.* 1999;7(3):189–198.

16. Wylie JD, Marchand LS, Burks RT. Etiologic factors that lead to failure after primary anterior cruciate ligament surgery. *Clin Sports Med.* 2017;36(1):155–172. https://doi.org/10.1016/j.csm.2016.08.007.

17. Dejour D, Kuhn ADH. Tibial deflexion osteotomy and chronic anterior laxity: a series of 22 cases. *Rev Chir Orthop.* 1998;84:28–29.

18. Butler DL, Noyes FR, Grood ES. Ligamentous restraints to anterior-posterior drawer in the human knee. A biomechanical study. *J Bone Jt Surg Am.* 1980;62(2):259–270.

19. Wordeman SC, Quatman CE, Kaeding CC, Hewett TE. In vivo evidence for tibial plateau slope as a risk factor for anterior cruciate ligament injury: a systematic review and meta-analysis. *Am J Sports Med.* 2012;40(7):1673–1681. https://doi.org/10.1177/0363546512442307.

20. Christensen JJ, Krych AJ, Engasser WM, Vanhees MK, Collins MS, Dahm DL. Lateral tibial posterior slope is increased in patients with early graft failure after anterior cruciate ligament reconstruction. *Am J Sports Med.* 2015;43(10):2510–2514. https://doi.org/10.1177/0363546515597664.

21. Yamaguchi KT, Cheung EC, Markolf KL, et al. Effects of anterior closing wedge tibial osteotomy on anterior cruciate ligament force and knee kinematics. *Am J Sports Med.* 2017:363546517736767. https://doi.org/10.1177/0363546517736767.

22. Harner CD, Giffin JR, Dunteman RC, Annunziata CC, Friedman MJ. Evaluation and treatment of recurrent instability after anterior cruciate ligament reconstruction. *Instr Course Lect.* 2001;50:463–474. http://www.ncbi.nlm.nih.gov/pubmed/11372347.

23. Drez DJ, DeLee J, Holden JP, Arnoczky S, Noyes FR, Roberts TS. Anterior cruciate ligament reconstruction using bone-patellar tendon-bone allografts. A biological and biomechanical evaluation in goats. *Am J Sports Med.* 1991;19(3):256–263. https://doi.org/10.1177/036354659101900308.

24. Salmon L, Russell V, Musgrove T, Pinczewski L, Refshauge K. Incidence and risk factors for graft rupture and contralateral rupture after anterior cruciate ligament reconstruction. *Arthrosc J Arthrosc Relat Surg.* 2005;21(8):948–957. https://doi.org/10.1016/j.arthro.2005.04.110.

25. Shelbourne KD, Gray T, Haro M. Incidence of subsequent injury to either knee within 5 years after anterior cruciate ligament reconstruction with patellar tendon autograft. *Am J Sports Med.* 2009;37(2):246–251. https://doi.org/10.1177/0363546508325665.

26. Lundquist RB, Matcuk GR, Schein AJ, et al. Posteromedial corner of the knee: the neglected corner. *Radiographics.* 2014;35(4):1123–1137.

27. Noyes FR, Barber-Westin SD, Hewett TE. High tibial osteotomy and ligament reconstruction for varus angulated anterior cruciate ligament-deficient knees. *Am J Sport Med.* 2000;28(3):282–296. https://doi.org/10.1177/036354659302100102.

28. Rossi R, Bonasia DE, A A. The role of high tibial osteotomy in the varus knee. *J Am Acad Orthop Surg.* 2011;19(10):590–599.

29. Hinterwimmer SMJ. Combination of ACL-replacement and high tibial osteotomy. *Oper Orthop Traumatol.* 2014;26(1):43–55.

30. Trojani C, Elhor H, Carles M, Boileau P. Anterior cruciate ligament reconstruction combined with valgus high tibial osteotomy allows return to sports. *Orthop Traumatol Surg Res.* 2014;100(2):209–212. https://doi.org/10.1016/j.otsr.2013.11.012.

31. Zhang H, Sun Y, Han X, et al. Simultaneous reconstruction of the anterior cruciate ligament and medial collateral ligament in patients with chronic ACL-MCL lesions. *Am J Sports Med.* 2014;42(7):1675–1681. https://doi.org/10.1177/0363546514531394.

32. Bollier MSP. Anterior cruciate ligament and medial collateral ligament injuries. *J Knee Surg.* 2014;27(5):359–368.

33. Kane PW, Wascher J, Dodson CC, Hammoud S, Cohen SB, Ciccotti MG. Anterior cruciate ligament reconstruction with bone-patellar tendon-bone autograft versus allograft in skeletally mature patients aged 25 years or younger. *Knee Surg Sport Traumatol Arthrosc.* 2016;24(11):3627–3633. https://doi.org/10.1007/s00167-016-4213-z.

34. Wright RW. Effect of graft choice on the outcome of revision anterior cruciate ligament reconstruction in the multicenter ACL revision study (MARS) cohort. *Am J Sports Med.* 2014;42(10):2301–2310. https://doi.org/10.1177/0363546514549005.

35. Jackson DW, Windler GESTE. Intraarticular reaction associated with the use of freeze-dried, ethylene oxide-sterilized bone-patella tendon-bone allografts in the reconstruction of the anterior cruciate ligament. *Am J Sport Med.* 1990;18(1):1–10.

36. Roberts TS, Drez DMW. Anterior cruciate ligament reconstruction using freeze-dried, ethylene oxide-sterilized, bone-patellar tendon-bone allografts. Two year results in thirty-six patients. *Am J Sports Med.* 1991;19(1):35–41.

37. Lamblin CJ, Waterman BR, Lubowitz JH. Anterior cruciate ligament reconstruction with autografts compared with non-irradiated, non-chemically treated allografts. *Arthrosc J Arthrosc Relat Surg.* 2013;29(6):1113–1122. https://doi.org/10.1016/j.arthro.2013.01.022.

38. Wei J, Yang HB, Qin JB, Yang TB. A meta-analysis of anterior cruciate ligament reconstruction with autograft compared with nonirradiated allograft. *Knee.* 2015;22(5):372–379. https://doi.org/10.1016/j.knee.2014.06.006.

39. Burrus MT, Werner BC, Crow AJ, et al. Increased failure rates after anterior cruciate? Ligament reconstruction with soft-tissue autograft-allograft hybrid grafts. *Arthroscopy.* 2015;31(12):2342–2351. https://doi.org/10.1016/j.arthro.2015.06.020.

40. Stein DA, Hunt SA, Rosen JE, Sherman OH. The incidence and outcome of patella fractures after anterior cruciate ligament reconstruction. *Arthroscopy.* 2002;18(6):578–583. https://doi.org/10.1053/jars.2002.30658.

41. Janssen RPA, van der Velden MJF, Pasmans HLM, Sala HAGM. Regeneration of hamstring tendons after anterior cruciate ligament reconstruction. *Knee Surg Sport Traumatol Arthrosc.* 2013;21(4):898–905. https://doi.org/10.1007/s00167-012-2125-0.

42. McRae S, Leiter J, McCormack R, Old J, MacDonald P. Ipsilateral versus contralateral hamstring grafts in anterior cruciate ligament reconstruction: a prospective randomized trial. *Am J Sports Med.* 2013;41(11):2492–2499. https://doi.org/10.1177/0363546513499140.

43. Wilk KE, Andrews JR, Clancy WG. Quadriceps muscular strength after removal of the central third patellar tendon for contralateral anterior cruciate ligament reconstruction surgery: a case study. *J Orthop Sports Phys Ther.* 1993;18(6):692–697. https://doi.org/10.2519/jospt.1993.18.6.692.

44. Shelbourne KD, Beck MB, Gray T. Anterior cruciate ligament reconstruction with contralateral autogenous patellar tendon graft: evaluation of donor site strength and subjective results. *Am J Sports Med.* 2015;43:648–653. https://doi.org/10.1177/0363546514560877.

45. Forkel P, Petersen W. Anatomic reconstruction of the anterior cruciate ligament with the autologous quadriceps tendon. Primary and revision surgery. *Oper Orthop Traumatol.* 2014;26(1):30–42. https://doi.org/10.1007/s00064-013-0261-4.

46. Laidlaw MS, Buyukdogan K, Werner BC, Miller MD. Management of bone deficiency in revision anterior cruciate ligament reconstruction. *Ann Jt.* 2017;5:1–12. https://doi.org/10.21037/aoj.2017.06.12.

47. Cooperman JM, Riddle DL, Rothstein JM. Reliability and validity of judgments of the integrity of the anterior cruciate ligament of the knee using the Lachman's test. *Phys Ther.* 1990;70(4):225–233. https://doi.org/10.1093/ptj/70.4.225.

48. Forsythe B, Saltzman BM, Cvetanovich GL, et al. Dial test: unrecognized predictor of anterior cruciate ligament deficiency. *Arthrosc J Arthrosc Relat Surg.* 2017;33(7):1375–1381. https://doi.org/10.1016/j.arthro.2017.01.043.

49. Rubinstein RA, Shelbourne KD, McCarroll JR, VanMeter CD, Rettig AC. The accuracy of the clinical examination in the setting of posterior cruciate ligament injuries. *Am J Sports Med.* 1994;22(4):550–557. https://doi.org/10.1177/036354659402200419.

50. Boyer P, Djian P, Christel P, Paoletti X, Degeorges R. Reliability of the KT-1000 arthrometer (Medmetric) for measuring anterior knee laxity: comparison with Telos in 147 knees. *Rev Chir Orthop Réparatrice L'appareil Mot.* 2004;90(8):757–764. http://www.ncbi.nlm.nih.gov/pubmed/15711494.

51. van Eck CF, Loopik M, van den Bekerom MP, Fu FH, Kerkhoffs GMMJ. Methods to diagnose acute anterior cruciate ligament rupture: a meta-analysis of instrumented knee laxity tests. *Knee Surg Sport Traumatol Arthrosc.* 2013;21(9):1989–1997. https://doi.org/10.1007/s00167-012-2246-5.

52. Di Stasi SL, Logerstedt D, Gardinier ES, Snyder-Mackler L. Gait patterns differ between ACL-reconstructed athletes who pass return-to-sport criteria and those who fail. *Am J Sports Med.* 2013;41(6):1310–1318. https://doi.org/10.1177/0363546513482718.

53. Moore SL. Imaging the anterior cruciate ligament. *Orthop Clin N Am.* 2002;33(4):663–674.

54. Gwathmey FW, Tompkins MA, Gaskin CM, Miller MD. Can stress radiography of the knee help characterize posterolateral corner injury? *Clin Orthop Relat Res.* 2012;470:768–773. https://doi.org/10.1007/s11999-011-2008-6.

55. Marchant MH, Willimon SC, Vinson E, Pietrobon R, Garrett WE, Higgins LD. Comparison of plain radiography, computed tomography, and magnetic resonance imaging in the evaluation of bone tunnel widening after anterior cruciate ligament reconstruction. *Knee Surg Sports Traumatol Arthrosc.* 2010;18(8):1059–1064. https://doi.org/10.1007/s00167-009-0952-4.

56. Meuffels DE, Potters JW, Koning AHJ, Brown Jr CH, Verhaar JAN, Reijman M. Visualization of postoperative anterior cruciate ligament reconstruction bone tunnels: reliability of standard radiographs, CT scans, and 3D virtual reality images. *Acta Orthop.* 2011;82(6):699–703. https://doi.org/10.3109/17453674.2011.623566.

57. Chahla J, Dean CS, Cram TR, et al. Two-stage revision anterior cruciate ligament reconstruction: bone grafting technique using an allograft bone matrix. *Arthrosc Tech.* 2016;5(1):e189–e195. https://doi.org/10.1016/j.eats.2015.10.021.

58. George MS, Dunn WR, Spindler KP. Current concepts review: revision anterior cruciate ligament reconstruction. *Am J Sports Med.* 2006;34(12):2026–2037. https://doi.org/10.1177/0363546506295026.

59. Thomas NP, Kankate R, Wandless F, Pandit H. Revision anterior cruciate ligament reconstruction using a 2-stage technique with bone grafting of the tibial tunnel. *Am J Sports Med.* 2005;33(11):1701–1709. https://doi.org/10.1177/0363546505276759.

60. Bach BR, Provencher MT. ACL surgery: how to get it right the first time and what to do if it fails. *J Sports Sci Med.* 2010;9(3):527.

61. Schulz AP, Götze S, Schmidt HGK, Jürgens C, Faschingbauer M. Septic arthritis of the knee after anterior cruciate ligament surgery: a stage-adapted treatment regimen. *Am J Sports Med.* 2007;35:1064–1069. https://doi.org/10.1177/0363546507299744.

62. Uchida R, Toritsuka Y, Mae T, Kusano M, Ohzono K. Healing of tibial bone tunnels after bone grafting for staged revision anterior cruciate ligament surgery: a prospective computed tomography analysis. *Knee.* 2016;23(5):830–836. https://doi.org/10.1016/j.knee.2016.04.012.

63. Werner BC, Gilmore CJ, Hamann JC, et al. Revision anterior cruciate ligament reconstruction: results of a single-stage approach using allograft dowel bone grafting for femoral defects. *J Am Acad Orthop Surg.* 2016;24(8):581–587. https://doi.org/10.5435/JAAOS-D-15-00572.

64. Bedi A, Allen A. Procedure 30: Revision anterior cruciate ligament reconstruction. In: Terry M, Reider B, Provencher M, eds. *Operative Techniques: Sports Medicine Surgery.* Philadelphia: Elsevier; 2010:487–514.

65. Wilde J, Bedi A, Altchek DW. Revision anterior cruciate ligament reconstruction. *Sports Health.* 2014;6(6):504–518. https://doi.org/10.1177/1941738113500910.

66. Mall N. Revision ACL reconstruction, indications and techniques. In: Marx R, ed. New York: Springer-Verlag; 2014.

67. Weiler A, Hoffmann RFG, Bail HJ, Rehm O, Südkamp NP. Tendon healing in a bone tunnel. Part II: histologic analysis after biodegradable interference fit fixation in a model of anterior cruciate ligament reconstruction in sheep. *Arthroscopy.* 2002;18(2):124–135. https://doi.org/10.1053/jars.2002.30657.

68. Colvin A, Sharma C, Parides M, Glashow J. What is the best femoral fixation of hamstring autografts in anterior cruciate ligament reconstruction? A meta-analysis. *Clin Orthop Relat Res.* 2011;469:1075–1081. https://doi.org/10.1007/s11999-010-1662-4.

69. Brand JC, Nyland J, Caborn DNM, Johnson DL. Soft-tissue interference fixation: bioabsorbable screw versus metal screw. *Arthrosc J Arthrosc Relat Surg.* 2005;21(8):911–916. https://doi.org/10.1016/j.arthro.2005.05.009.

70. Shen C, Jiang S-D, Jiang L-S, Dai L-Y. Bioabsorbable versus metallic interference screw fixation in anterior cruciate ligament reconstruction: a meta-analysis of randomized controlled trials. *Arthroscopy.* 2010;26(5):705–713. https://doi.org/10.1016/j.arthro.2009.12.011.

71. Anbari A, Bach B. Revision anterior cruciate ligament reconstruction. In: Cole BKSJ, ed. *Surgical Techniques of the Shoulder, Elbow, and Knee in Sports Medicine.* Philadelphia: Elsevier/Saunders; 2008:647–659.

72. Wright R, Spindler K, Huston L, et al. Revision ACL reconstruction outcomes: MOON cohort. *J Knee Surg.* 2011;24(4):289–294. https://doi.org/10.1055/s-0031-1292650.

73. Lefevre N, Klouche S, Mirouse G, Herman S, Gerometta A, Bohu Y. Return to sport after primary and revision anterior cruciate ligament reconstruction: a prospective comparative study of 552 patients from the FAST cohort. *Am J Sports Med.* 2016:363546516660075. https://doi.org/10.1177/0363546516660075.

74. Wright RW, Gill CS, Chen L, et al. Outcome of revision anterior cruciate ligament reconstruction: a systematic review. *J Bone Joint Surg Am.* 2012;94(6):531–536. https://doi.org/10.2106/JBJS.K.00733.

75. Ding DY, Zhang AL, Allen CR, et al. Subsequent surgery after revision anterior cruciate ligament reconstruction: rates and risk factors from a multicenter cohort. *Am J Sports Med.* 2017;45(9):2068–2076. https://doi.org/10.1177/0363546517707207.

76. Vaughn ZD, Schmidt J, Lindsey DP, Dragoo JL. Biomechanical evaluation of a 1-stage revision anterior cruciate ligament reconstruction technique using a structural bone void filler for femoral fixation. *Arthrosc J Arthrosc Relat Surg.* 2009;25(9):1011–1018. https://doi.org/10.1016/j.arthro.2009.04.068.

77. Tse BK, Vaughn ZD, Lindsey DP, Dragoo JL. Evaluation of a one-stage ACL revision Technique using bone void filler after cyclic loading. *Knee.* 2012;19(4):477–481. https://doi.org/10.1016/j.knee.2011.06.013.

CHAPTER 9

Anterior Cruciate Ligament Rehabilitation and Return to Play

SETH BLEE, MSPT, DPT, CFMT, CSCS

INTRODUCTION

As the previous chapters have focused on surgical interventions for the management of patients after anterior cruciate ligament (ACL) rupture, this chapter will focus on the rehabilitation and eventual return to play for these athletes. Patients who do not undergo surgical reconstruction will be briefly addressed as well; however, the majority of the focus will be on those athletes who do opt for surgical reconstruction of their ruptured ACL.

Just as no two injuries are exactly alike, no two surgeries are exactly alike, and therefore no two rehabilitation programs will be exactly alike. This chapter will address common concepts of ACL rehabilitation; however, the clinician must be acutely aware that this is not overly prescriptive and clinical judgement and experience, as well as patient response and patient values, must play a critical role in the rehabilitation program.

Evidence-based medicine (EBM) has been described as a three-legged stool,[1] with all three legs being of equal value when selecting appropriate interventions. These three components of EBM include utilizing the best clinical evidence available from the literature, combined with clinical experience and patient values. Relying too heavily on any one of these three components can result in a less than ideal outcome and can lead to falling short of obtaining the best results. This chapter will highlight key findings from the most current literature available while building on many years of clinical experience and patient interactions.

Orthopedic physicians who perform ACL surgeries will all agree that proper rehabilitation plays an essential role in maximizing the benefits of the surgery and maximizing the potential for a full recovery for the patient. Even the most skilled surgeon coupled with the most compliant and motivated patient will not be successful if the rehabilitation team does not utilize the best treatment interventions and the best clinical judgement. A major part of the successful rehabilitation of an athlete status post ACL reconstruction (ACLR) is the communication among the physical therapist, orthopedic surgeon, athletic trainers (when involved), and the patient. Clear expectations and goals are essential and must be developed among this group.

In the previous chapters, patient selection, concomitant injuries, options for graft selection, and variability of surgical interventions have been discussed. With such a large number of variables, it is critical for the physical therapist who is leading the rehabilitation program to communicate clearly with the referring physician. As will be discussed, the surgical procedure and the presence of additional injuries/interventions will have a major impact on the rehabilitation protocol and clinicians must be acutely aware of these issues as they begin working with the athlete. Part of the initial communication between the therapist and the surgeon should be a clear understanding on which graft was selected and the rationale behind the decision. The graft selection will have a significant impact on the focus of the rehabilitation and will give the therapist information on key things to look out for and about exercises that should and should not be included early in the program. Concomitant injuries must also be communicated with the therapist. As will be discussed later in this chapter, the presence of other injuries such as ruptures of the medial collateral ligament (MCL), lateral collateral ligament, posterior cruciate ligament (PCL), and medial or lateral menisci, as well as any significant bone bruising or soft tissue damage, will all impact the rehabilitation program and the rate at which an athlete can progress.

Many patients with ACL injury have setbacks and many actually fail in their recovery.[2] Failure of rehabilitation may be defined as suffering an additional tear and having the graft rupture, or it may be defined in the athletic population as not being able to return to the previous level of play. Key reasons for failed surgery/rehabilitation include technical failure of the surgery, including poor graft fixation, poor graft selection for a given patient, damage to the secondary restraints of the knee, poor lower extremity (LE) alignment predisposing an athlete to reinjury, persistent strength imbalances, and additional trauma to the recovering leg. Although some of these reasons do not pertain to the physical therapist and the rehabilitation team, it is critical to address all the potential reasons mentioned earlier, which can be managed by skilled therapy and appropriate interventions.

ALIGNMENT AND MECHANICAL CONCERNS

Research has consistently shown that certain alignments of the LEs can predispose athletes to ACL ruptures.[3] Often, athletes who have suffered an ACL rupture and completed a rehabilitation program will be discharged from treatment and cleared to return to their respective athletic activities without addressing these issues, which can continue to predispose them to injury or reinjury. Literature has demonstrated that there is a high reinjury rate (up to 30%) in female athletes within their first 6 months of returning to play. This may involve the same side or the contralateral side that frequently demonstrates the same alignment concerns that predisposed the athlete to injury in the first place.[4]

Certain static alignments have been shown to increase the risk of ACL injury, particularly in female athletes.[5] One of these risk factors is a large Q angle (measured from the anterosuperior iliac spine of the pelvis to the middle of the patella and down to the midpoint of the ankle) associated with female athletes having wider hips than male athletes. Although this bony alignment may not be modifiable, there are other coexisting issues that can be addressed. Typically, these female athletes will also have a higher amount of hip and pelvic internal rotation, increased genu valgus (knock-knee), and rear and midfoot compensations that cause collapsing of the medial longitudinal arch of the foot. Additionally, females have been shown to have increased laxity, particularly in rotational movements that stress the ACL, as compared with their male counterparts.[6] There is also an increase in the anterior tilt of the pelvis and an increase in the lordosis of the lumbar spine, both of which can impact efficient activation and firing of the core musculature. It is up to the therapist to manage these partially modifiable alignment dysfunctions in order to best maintain the health of the athlete and minimize the risk of reinjuring the repaired side or injuring the contralateral side. Regardless of the specifics of a surgeon's protocol, these mechanical issues can and should be addressed very early on in the rehabilitation of these athletes to optimize their potential for recovery and return to play.

NEUROMUSCULAR CONCERNS

In addition to bony alignment issues, female athletes often also present with strength imbalances and deficits that will need to be addressed as part of a successful program. Female athletes, particularly those with the dysfunctional alignment mentioned earlier, have certain imbalance that can also predispose them to injury of their knees, particularly their ACLs. These athletes often demonstrate weakness in their hip abductors and hip external rotators and an imbalance in their hamstrings relative to their quadriceps.[5] The timing of activation, particularly of the hamstrings relative to the quadriceps, has also shown to be different in females and males. As a result, attention should be given in the rehabilitation program to focus on training activation of the hamstrings and cocontraction of the entire LE musculature to best prevent injuries.[5] Strategies for this training will be discussed later in this chapter when discussing the key components of injury prevention programs. Strengthening of the muscles mentioned earlier must be a vital part of the rehabilitation program in order to best mitigate the risk factors for reinjury in these athletes.

MOTOR CONTROL

There have been well-documented differences in jumping and landing mechanics between female and male athletes that also play a role in the higher incidence of females sustaining knee injuries. The position of the knee when cutting and landing in female athletes tends to be in less knee flexion, leading to decreased activation of the hamstring muscles and therefore puts a higher demand on the ACL during athletics.[5] This must also be addressed as part of the later stages of the rehabilitation program and will be addressed later in the chapter.

While no one variable can be responsible for the higher prevalence of ACL injuries in female athletes compared with males, the statistics are definitely concerning. In multiple studies, female athletes have been consistently shown to suffer ACL ruptures at rates between six and eight times higher than their male counterparts. Although some of these risk factors may not be modifiable (smaller ACLs, laxity associated with hormonal changes in the menstrual cycle, wider pelvises, and increased Q angles), the contributing hip and foot alignment, muscle imbalances, and movement strategies mentioned earlier must be part of a thorough rehabilitation program for these athletes.

POSTOPERATIVE MANAGEMENT

Although most orthopedic surgeons' postoperative protocols will vary among the specifics, there are some general commonalities and themes that are shared among the majority. The key areas that may differ include weight-bearing status, use of bracing in the initial phases, range of motion (ROM) restrictions, use of continuous passive motion (CPM), and the type of wound closures used, which will impact wound care and scar management. All these variables make communication and understanding of surgical interventions a critical component of a successful rehabilitation program. In the following section, common interventions and guidelines will be presented for each phase of rehabilitation, but it is critical that the treating therapist remains in contact with the surgeon and modifies as needed throughout the program based on physician concerns about graft integrity, additional involved structures, and most importantly, patient response. Protocols should be used as guidelines to ensure protection of healing tissues but should not be viewed as overly prescriptive and standardized for all athletes. Rehabilitation of ACLRs in isolation will be addressed first followed by a discussion of key modifications when there are additional injuries and surgical procedures such as additional ligamentous repair, meniscal debridement or repair, microfractures, and in rare cases, LE fractures.

Early Rehabilitation (0–2 weeks)

While physicians differ in when they allow patients to begin physical therapy, it has been shown to be beneficial to start therapy as soon as possible. It is recommended that patients always schedule their physical therapy as soon as they schedule their surgery to minimize any delay in starting their rehabilitation due to therapist availability. With isolated ACLRs nearly always being done as outpatient procedures, the discussion of the rehabilitation program will start with outpatient physical therapy.

Ambulation status

In the early phases, many patients who have had isolated reconstruction of their ACL should be weight bearing as tolerated (WBAT), regardless of the graft selection. Patients should ambulate with bilateral crutches to avoid excessive compensations due to pain and inability to fully bear the weight on the involved leg. Often, patients are immobilized in braces that may be locked in extension for the first week, which will further impact ambulation status. The postoperative use of bracing is highly variable and is based on physician preference and concerns about stability of

the surrounding structures. Braces are generally used to prevent any anterior translation of the tibia on the femur, which may occur due to weakness of the surrounding dynamic stabilizers after operation. If a brace is unlocked allowing for knee flexion, or no brace is worn after operation, ambulation should still be WBAT during this early phase to protect the graft, to decrease stress on the surrounding tissues, and to minimize gait deviations. For patients who undergo meniscal repairs or MCL repairs along with ACLR, ambulation is generally limited to WBAT with a brace locked in extension for the first 4 weeks after operation.

Wound care

The techniques and devices used for closure of the wound are highly variable. It is the responsibility of the treating therapist to regularly inspect the wound for any obvious signs of infection, for excessive drainage, and for any other signs of impaired healing. Scar management will become a critical intervention but should not begin until the wound has adequately healed to avoid opening of the surgical site. If there are any concerns with tissue or wound healing, this must be communicated with the physician. The wound can be covered with Steri-Strips, bandages, ace wraps, etc. It is recommended to remove any unnecessary bandages and wraps that may interfere with the ability to move the knee and can limit the effect of cryotherapy.

Early range of motion

The most critical range to regain early in the rehabilitation protocol is full knee extension. This is often difficult because of the presence of edema, but treatment should focus on restoring this ROM as early as possible to prevent scarring down of tissues and to promote normal biomechanics of the knee joint for walking. In most cases, the goal of full extension should be achieved within the first 2 weeks and the physician should be notified if there are significant limitations to knee extension. Strategies should include ROM and soft tissue mobilization (STM) to both the posterior soft tissues (gastroc, soleus, popliteus, hamstring) and the quadriceps. There are controversies regarding whether or not to push for hyperextension, particularly in the hypermobile female athlete. It is generally accepted to work toward matching the contralateral limb, even if that knee goes into hyperextension, in order to decrease asymmetries.

Patellar mobilizations should also be included early in the rehabilitation program. Superior, inferior, medial, and lateral mobilizations should be performed by the therapist as well as taught to the patient to maintain mobility and decrease scar tissue formation. Care should be taken when performing inferior to superior mobilizations to avoid excessive stress to the surgical site, particularly when bone-tendon patellar-bone (BTB) grafts are used. In these cases, it is also important to perform STM to the medial and lateral borders of the patellar tendon to preserve tissue mobility.

Knee flexion ROM is also very important early on, and this will often be the most difficult movement for the patient. Frequent ROM should be performed to promote knee flexion to assist with circulation, tissue mobility, and activation of the hamstrings and to decrease fear of movement. Flexion ROM is generally only limited by patient tolerance, unless there are coexisting meniscal injuries and repairs that will often limit the flexion ROM to 90 degrees for the first 4 weeks.

Some physicians will still order the use of CPM machines to assist with early ROM of the knee. However, the long-term benefits of using CPM machines have not been validated, so the use of these devices is generally not justified and is rarely covered by insurance.[7] Assisted ROM can be performed with the contralateral leg instead of using a CPM machine.

The use of braces after operation also varies among physicians. Some will opt for limiting ROM early in the first 2 weeks to protect the limb, but this is done only when there are additional structures involved (MCL, meniscus). No studies have shown significant benefit to the use of braces to limit ROM in isolated ACLRs.[8]

Early exercises and modalities

Exercises should be started as soon as possible and should focus on promoting mobility of the surgically repaired leg. Initial exercises should include the following.
- Ankle pumps to promote circulation.
- Heel slides for knee flexion active ROM (AROM).
- Quadriceps isometrics (quad sets).
- Gluteal isometrics (glute sets).
- Hamstring isometrics (ham sets) in multiple angles. This may be delayed by 1–2 weeks with hamstring autografts due to pain.
- Straight leg raises (SLRs) may initially done with the braces locked in extension but can be progressed without them once the patient has adequate strength to avoid a quadriceps lag. SLRs can be done in all four planes for hip flexion, extension, abduction, and adduction (Adduction should be avoided when there is surgical repair of the MCL.).
- If weight bearing is allowed during this initial phase, patient should be encouraged to begin weight shifting onto the affected leg with upper extremity supports to train weight shifting and eventually full weight acceptance onto the leg to promote a return to full weight bearing.
- Electric stimulation (neuromuscular electric stimulation or the Russian setting) can be used to help better recruit muscle fibers for improved contraction of the quadriceps muscle early on. Using muscle stimulation can assist with contraction strength, particularly of the vastus medialis, which is generally very limited after surgery.[9] Any effusion on the knee will limit the ability of the quadriceps muscle to contract, so assisting the muscle recruitment with electric stimulation can be of additional benefit early on. The use of electric stimulation should not begin until the wound is closed and dry to decrease the risk of active bleeding.
- Cryotherapy is a vital component to manage edema of the involved LE. Frequent icing should be done several times per day in this early phase. It is most beneficial to combine cryotherapy with elevation to promote lymphatic drainage and when available, with vasopneumatic compression, to further assist with circulation.
- Blood flow restriction (BFR) therapy: The use of BFR therapy may be started early in the rehabilitation of the injured athlete, as long as edema is well controlled. BFR use will be covered under additional therapy considerations later in the chapter.

Additional manual therapy

Manual therapy techniques are highly variable among clinicians and will be impacted by the clinician's level of experience, continuing education background, treatment approach/philosophy, and confidence. The following manual therapy techniques should be included as part of a thorough rehabilitation program in order to maximize the benefit to the patient.
- ROM along with STM to soft tissues including gastroc, soleus, hamstrings, popliteus, and quadriceps. The research has clearly moved away from passive stretching in lieu of more beneficial active stretching techniques,[10] however, light passive stretching is appropriate in the early stages of rehabilitation.
- Joint mobilizations to the foot, ankle, hip, and pelvis as appropriate to begin to manage mechanical issues mentioned earlier and mitigate the risk of reinjury due to altered mechanical alignment. Common interventions should include mobilization of the calcaneus, talus, and navicular as needed to decrease internal rotation compensations of the foot, which may cause pronation and can contribute to

an increased valgus alignment of the knee. Pelvic and hip joint and STMs can also be implemented early on to address excessive internal rotation, which may also increase the valgus and adduction moment of the leg.

- Proprioceptive neuromuscular facilitation (PNF) techniques to train efficient firing of the core, pelvis, and hip should be included to begin to train appropriate integration of the LE and trunk.

Key components of the rehabilitation program

During this initial phase of therapy, communication between the patient and the therapist is vital. The therapist should outline the course of rehabilitation and set expectations for the patient. Compliance with the designated therapy program must be stressed if the athlete is to make a full recovery. Compliance with coming in for treatment must be stressed, and this typically involves treatment sessions for two to three times per week in most outpatient settings. With this plan of care, it must be stressed that the athlete's home exercise program (HEP) will be a critical component of the rehabilitation program, and compliance with the prescribed HEP will often dictate the success of the rehabilitation program. It is also important to discuss the long-term goals and the appropriate time frames for return to activity to best prepare the patient for the lengthy recovery process.

Second Phase of Rehabilitation (2–6 weeks)

All the ROM exercises, soft tissue and joint mobilizations, and manual therapy techniques mentioned in the initial phase should be continued in this next phase of rehabilitation.

Ambulation status

In isolated ACLR surgeries, by the 2-week mark, most patients are increasing their weight-bearing status and begin to wean off of crutches. This is generally done with a progression to one crutch (on the contralateral side) and then to no crutches as patients become able to demonstrate minimal gait deviations and are able to show good weight acceptance on the involved limb, with stride lengths and stance times close to equal to the uninvolved side. Brace wear continues to vary based on the physician, but in nearly all cases, patients will be free to ambulate with a brace unlocked. Many physicians will allow patients to discontinue the brace once their quadriceps strength is adequate to allow for SLRs without a lag. For ACLs combined with microfracture procedures, patients are often non–weight bearing for 4 weeks followed by a gradual return to weight-bearing status over the next 2–3 weeks.

Wound care

As the surgical wounds should be well healed by this time, scar tissue management should be included. This should be done with STM to the scar(s), cross-friction massage, and STM to the surrounding tissues. Patients can often be shown how to perform self-treatment of their scars and can also be provided information regarding appropriate topical ointments that can be used to help with scar healing.

Range of motion

ROM should be progressed throughout this phase, with full active extension being critical to achieve. Knee flexion AROM should also be progressed with STM of the quadriceps and hamstrings, continued patellar mobilizations, retrograde STM to manage edema, and light stretching focusing on active stretching (active elongation, hold-relax, and contract-relax) techniques. For patients who undergo meniscal repairs and/or MCL repairs, ROM is generally limited to 90 degrees for the first 4 weeks. Bracing in these scenarios often involve an extended knee, with the brace locked in extension for the first 4 weeks of ambulation as well.

Exercise additions

This will not be an all-inclusive list of exercises but some key guidelines and key exercises will be discussed. These are in addition to early exercises mentioned in the initial phase.

- Closed chain exercises (weight bearing): Most ACL rehabilitation programs will focus on closed chain exercises. This is done to train cocontraction of various muscle groups and to promote functional strengthening. It is always more functional to train muscles together because that is how the human body functions. When training in closed chain, there is integration of multiple joints and multiple muscle groups. In most cases, therapists should avoid training any muscles in isolation and should focus more on cocontractions, with an emphasis on functional training. This cocontraction promotes the best activation of the dynamic stabilizers and as such can decrease laxity of the knee. When performing closed chain exercises during this phase of rehabilitation, exercises should be kept from 0 to 60 degrees as much as possible to avoid the stress on the knee that occurs with deep knee flexion in weight-bearing positions.[11] This is particularly important with BTB grafts to avoid excessive stress to the healing patellar tendon. Varying types of contractions (isometric, concentric, and eccentric control) should be introduced as multiple ways to retrain the muscles for efficient functioning.

Common closed chain exercises include
- bridges (many variables with stable and unstable surfaces, double vs. single leg),
- use of stationary bicycles early on in this phase,
- mini squats (0–60 degrees),
- light leg press,
- terminal knee extension,
- small range step-ups (anterior and lateral to begin),
- initiate lunges in small ranges as tolerated,
- progression to the use of elliptical trainer in the later stages of this phase.
- Open chain exercises (non–weight bearing): Although not the focus of treatment, open chain exercises can be beneficial if they are done in protected ranges. Terminal extension of the knee should be avoided (final 30 degrees of extension), as it has been shown to create increased shear forces on the knee.[11]

Common open chain exercises include the following.
- Progression of SLRs in all four planes. Ankle weights can be added as able, but care must be taken to ensure adequate quadriceps strength evidenced by the absence of a lag. Performing adduction SLR should be cautioned in patients who also underwent MCL repairs.
- Hamstring curls—prone, seated, or standing. This can be implemented but caution should be taken with hamstring grafts (avoid if PCL reconstruction also has been undergone).
- Standing hip flexion, extension, abduction, and adduction. These can be done with resistance and can be performed bilaterally for incorporation of proprioceptive training if the athlete has adequate balance, trunk stability, and core activation. Resistance can be applied with elastic bands either at the proximal aspect of the upper leg to emphasize hip strengthening or more distally to focus more on balance reactions.
- Knee extensions can be incorporated but this should only be done in protected ranges (90–30 degrees). Any addition of resistance should be placed as far proximal on the tibia as possible to decrease shear forces on the knee. Although some protocols allow for knee extensions in this phase of rehabilitation, it is prudent and is recommended to wait until later in the rehabilitation progression (>12 weeks) to incorporate this exercise as needed. This exercise is also not recommended in this early phase with BTB grafts.

- Proprioceptive training should be started as soon as the patient is safe with weight bearing on the involved leg. There are benefits in incorporating proprioceptive exercises even earlier on the unaffected side. Research has shown that even short periods of inactivity and lack of use of an injured body part lead to changes in the sensory cortex of the brain.[12] It becomes critical to begin to both retrain the involved body part to better connect the segment to the brain and reinstitute efficient mapping on the homunculus.
  - Balance training may be done in a wide variety of ways. This training involves multiple stabilizers surrounding multiple joints and can be progressed as tolerated. Patients should always be guarded closely when adding new balance challenges and should be monitored for compensatory movement patterns. When performing standing balance exercises, the stance limb should always remain in slight knee flexion to better activate recruitment of the hamstrings. Equipment used can include resistance bands and unstable surfaces such as foam pads, rocker and wobble boards, and trampolines.
  - Stabilization and perturbation training can be performed manually by a therapist who is adept at noticing patient motor firing patterns and compensations.
  - PNF techniques aimed at the pelvis, trunk, and LE to retrain integration of the entire LE and to ensure efficient movement patterns should be included.
  - Core stabilization exercises are critical for stability and should be focused on maintaining stability around the pelvic girdle and the hips to promote efficient LE movement patterns and to avoid compensations due to trunk weakness.[13]
- Modalities
  - Cryotherapy should be continued to manage any effusion or edema.
  - Vasopneumatic compression can be done in isolation or can be combined with cryotherapy to assist in edema management.
  - Electric stimulation can be continued in this phase but should be weaned off once the patient is able to activate appropriate muscle contractions on his/her own.
  - BFR can be used and will be discussed later.

Subacute Phase (6–12 weeks)

During this phase, each of the abovementioned areas are progressed based on patient response. Weight bearing should be full without compensations, ROM should be equal to the nonsurgical side, soft tissues should continue to be managed with manual therapy, and mobilizations to proximal and distal segments to address alignment should be continued as needed.

Manual therapy should continue and scar tissue mobilization can become more aggressive to break up any restrictions along or around the scar. Patellar mobilizations, primarily from inferior to superior can also become more aggressive once the surgical site is completely healed. Additionally, soft tissue restrictions should continue to be managed throughout the quadriceps, hamstrings, gastroc, popliteus, adductors, and along the quadriceps/iliotibial band borders. Dry needling is often used in the therapy setting to manage soft tissue restrictions and is generally not recommended before 6 weeks of operation. Although the risk of infection is extremely low with dry needling, it is recommended to wait until the wound is fully closed and well healed, and even then, care should be taken not to introduce needling and skin disruptions right around the incision site. Needling can be very beneficial in managing soft tissue restrictions and trigger points throughout the quadriceps muscle, in particular, and can decrease anterior knee pain and improve knee flexion ROM by managing surrounding soft tissue mobility.[14]

As long as wounds are completely closed and remain dry and intact, walking in the water can be instituted to promote normal gait mechanics and to address weight-bearing deviations. Gravity-eliminated treadmills are also helpful during this phase, as they allow the therapist to guide the patient in efficient weight bearing and normal gait mechanics without the loading through the joint that may contribute to some of the gait deviations. In water or the gravity-eliminated environment, loads can be gradually increased to better simulate a normal walking condition on dry land.

During this next phase, exercises continue to be progressed to regain strength and balance throughout the lower body. Emphasis should continue to be on closed chain exercises for functional strengthening and for coactivation of various muscle groups. All exercises should remain pain free and should be closely monitored for proper form. Key exercises include the following.

- Squats can progress to weighted squats. ROM can gradually increase as the athlete approaches the later weeks of this phase. Maintaining the knees over or slightly behind the toes has been shown to decrease the stress on the ACL.[11]

- Lunges can include addition of weights but additional weight is likely not needed. Lunges can be performed on flat ground or on slide boards and can include multiple directions (forward, backward, lateral, diagonal). Focus should be on maintaining neutral LE alignment and avoiding valgus.
- With both squats and lunges, a slight forward tilt of the trunk increases hamstring activation and decrease anterior translation of the tibia.[11]
- Forward trunk bends including bilateral dead lifts, Romanian dead lifts, and hip hinges.
- Step-ups and step-downs can be introduced for closed chain concentric and eccentric control, primarily, of the quadriceps. Particular attention should be paid to any complaints of increased anterior knee pain, especially with BTB grafts. Proper form focused on pelvic and trunk control is vital when performing this exercise, as many patients tend to deviate into a valgus alignment of the knee and an internal rotation of the hip and pelvis.
- Additional resistance can be provided around the trunk, pelvis, or hips with many of these exercises to better activate a core stabilizing contraction and to target key areas of weakness such as hip internal rotators and abductors.
- Balance exercises should be an area of emphasis during this phase to continue to address proprioception and the neuroreflexive response.
- Manually resisted exercises by a skilled therapist are key in training appropriate motor responses. Therapists should use manual resistance to assess muscle imbalances, aberrant firing patterns, key areas of weakness or compensations, and the ability to perform varying types of contractions (isometric, concentric, and eccentric). This attention to detail is critical and can often be missed when using machines alone for resistance training. PNF manual resistance is particularly beneficial in evaluating different components of movements as well as evaluating and training how different muscles work together in combined movement patterns.

Graft strength

A key consideration during this phase of rehabilitation and recovery is the strength of the graft. Care must be taken to acknowledge the phases of tissue healing and understand that there is a period when the graft is being remodeled and incorporated into the body that will actually temporarily weaken the tensile strength. This is generally between 6 and 10 weeks.[15] This is imperative to discuss with patients, particularly with athletes, as this time often coincides with when pain has subsided and they begin to feel like they can do more stressful activities. The athlete must be educated on the biology of the healing tissue and to avoid additional stresses beyond what the therapist has allowed.

It has been shown that allografts are incorporated more slowly and less completely, so there will be inherently less ability.[16] As has been discussed in earlier chapters, the research currently does not support the use of allografts in young female athletes, as the failure rate of allografts has been shown to be significantly higher than both BTB and hamstring autografts.[17]

12–16 weeks

During this phase, the treatments mentioned earlier and the previous concepts discussed should continue to be progressed. Proprioceptive and strength training are continually progressed with some additional concepts introduced. Varying speeds of exercises can be incorporated, particularly for athletes who are in phasic dominant types of sports that require fast-twitch muscle contractions. Stability training can be progressed and should incorporate the entire body, including the upper extremities, as needed for the athlete's given sport or recreational activity.

Return to running and jumping

There is a great amount of variability when it comes to allowing an athlete to return to running and jumping activities. ROM should be equal to the uninvolved side and strength should be progressing to approach the other side as well. Effusion should no longer be present and the firing patterns of the quadriceps and hamstrings should be efficient. Most protocols will allow for a return to running and initiating plyometrics at the 12-week mark and this can be used as a guide; however, athlete's response to previous treatment and strength and neuromuscular control should be the deciding factor rather than time. Some protocols will allow running as early as 8 weeks status post ACLR, but it is very unusual to have a patient who has met all the requirements mentioned previously at that early stage. It is recommended that prior to initiating running the athlete have full AROM, especially into knee extension, efficient firing of the quadriceps, efficient eccentric control of both the hamstrings and the quadriceps, adequate push off of the ankle plantar flexors, and an overall LE strength of 70%–80% of the uninvolved limb.[18]

As running has been described as an alternate hopping on each leg, an athlete should be able to push off adequately on the involved leg to allow for efficient propulsion forward of their full body weight as needed

for hopping. The athlete also needs to have the balance and neuromuscular control to land on the involved leg without pain, loss of balance, or trunk compensations. Alternate hopping activities and single-limb stance with resistance should be incorporated prior to attempting running. Ground reaction forces and joint velocities are much higher during running than during these prerunning activities, so even these activities can be deceiving when gauging an athlete's readiness to return to running.[19]

When the athlete is able to begin running, a mini trampoline is a recommended way to start. This will decrease the ground reaction force and the stress to the knee. Another benefit of the mini trampoline is that it will encourage the athlete to maintain some amount of increased knee flexion with landing, which will facilitate activation of the hamstrings. As hamstrings are key dynamic stabilizers of the knee and act to prevent anterior translation of the tibia on the femur, increased activation of the hamstrings can help decrease the stress on the repaired ACL. An additional benefit will be that the trampoline will encourage athletes to stay more on their toes during both push off and landing, which limits the extensor stress on the joint.

Another activity that can be very helpful at training the coactivation of the involved leg is backward running. Backward running can be done as backpedaling in the clinic, on a field, or at slow speeds on a treadmill under close supervision. This will encourage the athlete to stay on the balls of the feet and keep the knees flexed to better recruit the hamstrings to protect the ACL. Maintaining a partial squat or hip hinge position will ensure activation of the hamstrings and the quadriceps to provide for cocontraction of the anterior and posterior muscle groups, enabling stability in the sagittal plane.

When available to the athlete, running in environments that are able to decrease the effect of gravity and ground reaction forces is recommended initially. Underwater treadmills and gravity-eliminated treadmills, such as the AlterG, are excellent ways to off-load some of the body weight and decrease stress while allowing for training of efficient running mechanics. Once efficient running mechanics are observed, body weight percentages can be increased to full body weight as tolerated. The high cost of this type of equipment makes it very rare in most rehabilitation clinics outside the professional sports setting. If full-body-weight running is done initially, the therapist must be acutely aware of the compensations and should train the athlete to minimize these deviations as much as possible.

Functionalization Phase (16 weeks to 6 months and Beyond)

During this later phase of recovery, the athlete enters the functionalization phase. Focused attention should be on higher level dynamic activities to prepare the athletes to return to their sports and recreational activities of choice. This phase should not be rushed and should last for at least 2–3 months to allow for neuromuscular education and functional training. Throughout this phase, as exercises and demands are increased, careful attention must be paid to ensure that the athlete does not experience any additional pain (often anterior knee pain occur with BTB grafts and hamstring pain with hamstring autografts). The athlete should also remain free from increased effusion or edema on the knee, which can limit efficient motor firing patterns. Key aspects to include in this phase are the introduction to sport and the activity–specific demands on the knee, including jumping, cutting, pivoting, and agility drills. Proprioceptive exercises and activities that refresh and restore efficient and appropriate movement patterns are the key to this phase. The gradual incorporation of these types of activities also help athletes to gradually build confidence and trust in the strength and stability of their surgically repaired leg. Another vital component of this later phase of rehabilitation is the incorporation of an ACL prevention program to mitigate the risk factors of reinjuring the surgically repaired leg as well as to decrease the chance of injuring the contralateral leg.

PREVENTION PROGRAMS

There are many different ACL prevention programs that have been developed to help mitigate the risk of ACL rupture, particularly in the female athlete. The key components of prevention programs should be used both in the prevention model and during the later stages of rehabilitation after surgery. The programs can help with retraining the athlete in efficient body mechanics and jumping/landing training. This will help with strengthening and retraining the athlete for return to play, as well as addressing any dysfunctions that may have initially predisposed the athlete to injury in the first place. Both legs will be included in this training to decrease the risk of not only reinjuring the affected leg but also injuring the contralateral leg.

As 80%–90% of noncontact ACL tears happen in individuals with hypermobility, primarily in hyperextension, it becomes critical to train both the limbs to avoid this high-risk position when performing athletic activities. Athletes should be trained to stay out of recurvatum as much as possible to better activate the hamstrings and to decrease the chance of an anterior shear force of the tibia on the femur.

A common component of prevention programs is the activation of the hamstrings and training the athlete to attain positions with increased knee flexion to prevent shear forces and to help stabilize the knee. The hamstring muscles are critical for dynamic stabilization of the knee and must be trained to remain active as much as possible. Hamstrings have been shown to reduce anterior translation of the tibia, but this is minimized when the knee is in complete extension. The hamstrings are best able to provide the stability assistance to the ACL when positioned in 15–30 degrees of knee flexion. Stability of the knee comes from both the static and dynamic forces working together. When performing a transitional movement that stresses the knee, the ligaments or static stabilizers initially stabilize the knee in the first 0–0.25 second. From 0.25 to 1.0 second after stress is introduced, the muscle or dynamic stabilizers activate to protect the knee. If the muscles are already active, the more likely that these dynamic stabilizers will be active to provide stability. With this in mind, maintaining slight knee flexion, particularly at times of impact or directional changes, is recommended to keep the knees flexed to better keep the hamstrings activated.

FEMALES VERSUS MALES

The question is often asked as to why women are at such a higher risk for ACL injuries than men. The reasons are multifactorial, and several theories have already been thoroughly addressed in the earlier sections of this book. Some of the common theories discussed involve structural reasons including wider pelvic bones producing increased Q angles, increased joint and ligamentous laxity, and a narrower intercondylar notch. In addition, there are hormonal factors associated with estrogen levels that produce increased joint laxity and decreased collagen strength. There are also training differences and strength differences that are evident between male and female athletes, some of which will be mentioned in the following.

As discussed earlier, the hamstrings are critical dynamic stabilizers of the knee and are best activated when maintaining a slightly flexed knee position, primarily with landing, cutting, and pivoting. Hamstring strength, power, and peak torque have been shown to be significantly weaker in females than in males. Studies have also found that there can be significant imbalances in hamstring activation between male and female athletes. Male athletes, in general, often demonstrate three times the activation of hamstrings upon landing than their female counterparts.[5] Female athletes have also been shown in multiple studies to have decreased hamstring activation and decreased protection of the knee against both anterior translation and rotational torsion during athletics as compared with their male counterparts.[20]

DO THESE PREVENTION PROGRAMS WORK?

In several studies conducted by Dr. Hewett, Dr. Noyes, and the Cincinnati Sports Medicine Institute, the prevention program used (Sportsmetrics) was found to make significant changes to strength, neuromuscular activation, and motor control when performed over a 6-week period. Results of these studies revealed an increased hamstring-to-quadriceps ratio (13% in the dominant side and 26% in the nondominant side), decreased landing forces (22%), decreased knee adduction moments (50%), increased hamstring power (44% on the dominant side and 21% on the nondominant side), and increased vertical jump height (10%). All these statistics showed that by training female athletes in an ACL prevention program, their risk factors for sustaining an ACL injury can be decreased to levels equal to those of their male counterparts.[5]

Many prevention programs have similar components and have been discussed in detail earlier in this book. The rehabilitation professional should include the components of addressing and managing LE alignment, training appropriate strength and the balance of anterior and posterior musculature, along with training motor control and proper mechanics for jumping, cutting, and higher agility movements needed during athletic activities. All the exercises and movements discussed in the prevention programs should be included in a thorough rehabilitation and return to play protocol. It is recommended that these be addressed after the athlete is able to run without any compensations and has demonstrated strength and balance within 85% of the contralateral limb. Owing to the potential laxity of allografts, some physicians will not recommend performing these jump training programs in athletes who have had allograft reconstructions.

BLOOD FLOW RESTRICTION

The American College of Sports Medicine (ACSM) has recommended that muscle should be stressed and exercised at loads greater than 70% of a one repetition maximum (1RM) for a person to gain strength and hypertrophy a muscle.[21] To maximize the benefits of an exercise program and obtain hypertrophy, muscles must be put under these relatively high amounts of stress. Obviously after a surgery, it is not possible and not at all safe to put that much load on a healing tissue. Regardless of the graft type, the newly constructed ACL graft should not be stressed at anywhere near those loads while it is in the healing phase. With this in mind, there has been a lot of research conducted to determine if there was a way to stress the body and get the hypertrophic response without putting such high levels of stress on the affected body part.[22,23]

One promising area of research has been in the field of BFR therapy. It has been shown that by exercising under conditions of restricted blood flow to muscles using significantly lighter loads (20% of 1RM), the body can receive the same metabolic benefits as it does when lifting with much heavier loads (80% 1RM). There are multiple theories that continue to be explored to attempt to explain why these strength gains are achieved. The following paragraphs will provide a brief introduction into the field of BFR therapy; however, it is highly recommended that any rehabilitation professional interested in learning more about this field of study should take additional classes on this topic before using it on their patients. The scientific theories and evidence behind BFR will be discussed briefly in the following paragraphs.

There are significant changes that occur in the body when lifting heavy weights. High-intensity exercises with heavy loads cause breakdown of muscle tissue to stimulate repair via protein synthesis. Low-level exercises, which are commonly done early in the postoperative therapy phase, do not break down tissue enough to stimulate protein synthesis needed for muscle hypertrophy to maximize strength gains. By exercising with low loads under conditions of decreased oxygen availability, the body switches from an aerobic to an anaerobic pathway that can trigger the same protein synthesis as is seen with heavy lifting. This is promising in the rehabilitation phase, as it becomes possible to receive the same metabolic effects experienced with heavy lifting when the patient performs much lighter lifting under conditions of restricted blood flow.

The basis for how this happens will be discussed briefly to give the clinician a baseline understanding as to why this type of training can be effective.

When heavy lifting is performed, the body switches from slow-twitch oxidative muscle fibers to fast-twitch anaerobic fibers. This anaerobic exercise leads to the accumulation of both lactate and hydrogen ions in the muscle tissue. This buildup of lactic acid triggers the release of human growth hormone (HGH) from the pituitary gland. This in turn triggers the release of insulinlike growth factor 1 (name) that stimulates protein synthesis and muscle hypertrophy. Levels of lactate accumulated in the blood has been shown to be similar between the group that used BFR with 20% 1RM and the high-intensity training group using 80% 1RM.[24] High-intensity training causes a significant increase in the levels of HGH in the body, but it has been shown that the group that exercised with lighter loads (20% 1RM) had a 290% increase in HGH levels compared with baseline and a 1.7 times increase compared with the high-intensity group.[22] Additionally, the release of HGH has also been shown to trigger collagen synthesis, which can be an additional benefit of BFR training to facilitate remodeling of collagen after a trauma or surgery.

Myostatin is a human genetic component that blocks the synthesis of protein. It helps humans to self-regulate and avoid putting on muscle mass every time physical exertion and tissue breakdown occurs, as it is metabolically costly to build and sustain increased muscle mass. Studies have shown that in just 9 weeks of heavy resistance training (85% of 1RM), there is a downregulation of myostatin, which allows the body to put on additional muscle mass.[25] BFR training with low loads (20% of 1RM) have been shown to have comparable effects of myostatin regulation as heavy loads.[25]

An additional theory explaining the strength gains seen with BFR is the muscle activation theory. As muscles build up lactate, the contraction of the motor units of those specific fibers affected is inhibited. In order to continue to exercise, additional motor units need to be recruited to maintain muscle contraction. By exercising with BFR and low loads, the production of lactate has been shown to stimulate the recruitment of additional motor units and thereby increasing the number of fibers that are utilized during an exercise.[26]

With several different pathways likely contributing to the benefits of exercising with BFR, this is a treatment modality that is gaining more and more acceptance as the research continues to show promising outcomes. It is becoming evident that exercising with lower loads with BFR is able to enhance the body's ability to synthesize protein and take this critical step in building strength without causing muscle fiber damage or putting undue stress on healing grafts and tissues.

CONCOMITANT INJURIES AND ADDITIONAL PROCEDURES

As was discussed in the acute management of patients in the postoperative phase, additional procedures will impact the rate of progression and the specifics of the protocol that should be followed. For example, when an ACL is combined with an MCL repair, there will inevitably be a prolonged period of decreased weight bearing, likely in a knee immobilizer to allow for proper healing of the MCL repair. When the ACL is coupled with a meniscal repair, there will also be decreased weight bearing initially, frequently coupled with a prolonged period of protected ROM to avoid undue stress on the repaired meniscus. Microfractures may also be performed in conjunction with the ACLR, particularly when the trauma of the injury also causes a significant enough shear force to cause damage to the surrounding cartilage on either the femoral condyles or the tibial plateau. When this procedure is done, athletes will likely also be non–weight bearing for an extended period to allow for healing and growth of the affected cartilage. Once the initial protective phase has been completed and the athlete is cleared to progress, he or she should advance as discussed earlier through similar progressions, with frequent communication with the surgeon.

NONSURGICAL CASES

Not all athletes who suffer a rupture of their ACL choose to have surgical reconstruction of the affected ligament. Some athletes and physicians opt for more conservative treatments and rely on strengthening the surrounding tissues, activity modifications, and pharmacologic treatments to manage the athlete's condition. In most cases, the younger the athlete and the higher the athlete's level of competition, the more likely that he or she will opt for a surgical reconstruction. For younger athletes who want to return to competing at high levels, research supports that surgical repair is the most successful option.[27] For those older or less competitive athletes who opt for nonoperative treatment, a thorough rehabilitation program is critical to maximize potential for recovery and for participation in athletics. This program should include addressing the mechanical and alignment issues mentioned earlier, the neuromuscular retraining of efficient motor firing and movement patterns, and the functional strengthening described earlier in this chapter. Strengthening should particularly focus on the hamstrings and their role in preventing anterior shearing of the tibia on the femur. This dynamic stabilizer of the knee will aid in the functioning of the impaired ACL and help to decrease stress on the knee that occurs from excessive anterior translation.

RETURN TO PLAY

One of the most difficult decisions that a rehabilitation team will make is when to clear an athlete to return to play. There are many variables to consider, including strength and balance relative to the unaffected leg, ratio of quadriceps to hamstring strength, agility and speed, performance of functional tests, isokinetic testing (when available), confidence levels, and activity requirements for the given activity. Even with the best data and the highest performance on these tests, deciding on when to return to play still comes down to an educated guess. Unfortunately, many practitioners base this decision primarily on the amount of time out of surgery rather than on objective measures and completion of standardized tests.[28] This important decision should not be made based on time alone and the athlete should always successfully complete an array of testing. The psychologic aspects of returning to play should also be taken into consideration and should be addressed by a qualified professional.

One key component that most physical therapists and physicians look to when assessing readiness to return to sport is the overall strength of the leg. A statistic that has often been referred to is the quadriceps-to-hamstring strength ratio.[28–31] As hamstrings are critical to provide dynamic stabilization to the knee, regaining and maximizing hamstring strength is crucial to protect the knee as athletes return to their given activities. However, relying too much on the quadriceps-to-hamstring ratio must be cautioned, as many athletes present with a favorable strength ratio at the expense of quadriceps strength. Quadriceps strength and control is also critical so it should not be overlooked when focusing on this strength ratio of anterior to posterior musculature.

Functional Strength Testing

There are almost as many functional tests to determine readiness to return to play as there are different protocols to follow postoperatively. There is no one test to determine when an athlete is ready to return to the field and the decision must be based on various factors. The athlete must be pain free without any edema or effusion on the knee, ROM should be equal to the uninvolved side, and strength should be between 85% and 90% of the uninvolved side. The athlete must also demonstrate good proprioception and kinesthetic

awareness and must have confidence in the leg's ability to withstand the challenges of the athlete's given sport or activity.

Some common functional strength assessments include the following.

- Ability to perform step-downs or single-leg squats with both eccentric and concentric control. These can be measured by the number of repetitions performed with adequate control in a 30-second period. The number of repetitions completed should be within 10% of the contralateral side.[32]
- Single-leg hops for distance (taking off and landing on the same foot), with the involved side covering >85% of the distance of the uninvolved.[33]
- Triple hop for distance, with the involved side covering >85% of the distance of the uninvolved.[34]
- A sequence of hops including a single hop for distance, a 6-m timed hop, a triple hop for distance, and crossover hops for distance.[33] Based on the results of these hops, dynamic knee stability can be quantified and compared with the unaffected leg.
- Single-leg forward, lateral, and crossover hops without loss of balance, while maintaining proper alignment of the LE.
- Single-leg squat or leg press test with weight pressed, with the involved side covering >85% of the uninvolved leg.
- Jumping, jump down tests, and repeated jumps can also be observed and video recorded for analysis to ensure proper LE tracking and alignment.
- Isokinetic strength testing can also be done to compare strength between one side and the other as well as to compare the quadriceps-to-hamstring ratio. Isokinetic testing has become less common because practitioners have favored more functional testing that theoretically should correlate better to the field of play.
- Sports-specific agility drills that should be tailored to meet the demands of each individual sport are required.
- Inclusion of a self-reported outcome questionnaire such as the Lower Extremity Functional Scale or the Lysholm outcome tool can also be helpful in assessing perception of functional capabilities.

REALITY CHECK

Less than 60% of patients make a full recovery, as measured by the ability to return to sports at the same level of play.[2] A high percentage of athletes do not return to the same level, this could be due to physical reasons, psychologic reasons, motivational issues, or simply choosing to give up playing the sport at the same high level. In studies that have looked at the general population and their return to play, results have shown that 82% of recreational athletes are able to return to some level of sports participation, 63% return to their preinjury levels of participation, and 44% return to competitive sports at their final follow-up.[35] In professional athletes, studies have shown that between 63% and 80% of National Football League players have been able to return to participate in professional football games,[36] 78% of National Basketball Association players were able to return to professional basketball games,[37] and 88% of Major League Baseball players were able to return to professional baseball games.[38] Many of these studies also tracked performance measures in a large percentage of these players and showed a decline in their performance metrics and their playing time after injury.

Unfortunately, many athletes who do return to sports suffer reinjury when attempting to return before the injured leg is ready to support the demands that come with athletics. These relatively high rates of reinjury have been particularly significant in female athletes. In studies examining the high risks of reinjury,[2] females were found to have between 4% and 6% rate of retear of the involved ACL and between 7% and 12% tear rate of the contralateral ACL for a combined reinjury rate between 12% and 20%. This is compared with 4.1% rate on the ipsilateral leg, 3.7% on the contralateral leg, and a total of 8% reinjury rate in male athletes. These rates of reinjury were highest in the younger population (17.4% in those female athletes younger than 18 years). Other studies have seen overall reinjury rates as high as 32% in athletes under 18 years of age.[40] Studies have also examined multiple factors to determine any key indicators that may predispose athletes to reinjury, and the only predictor of a second ACL injury was an earlier return to sports.[40]

Traditionally, strength deficits have persisted well after athletes have returned to play following ACLR surgery. Over the past 25 years, athletes have averaged 75%–85% strength in the affected leg compared with that of the unaffected leg based on isokinetic testing at 6 months after operation. This shows that even at 6 months after surgery, there is still a 15%–25% strength deficit, primarily due to quadriceps weakness. Knee extensor moments have also been shown to be as high as 35% from 6 to 15 months after surgery during high-level athletic activities such as running, jumping, and hopping. This asymmetric LE strength has

been seen particularly when evaluating the eccentric control of the LE after an ACLR.[41,42] This weakness has been shown to be due to muscle atrophy as opposed to central inhibition or neuromuscular activation deficits, even up to 6 months after surgery.[43] Furthermore, adolescent patients have demonstrated strength deficits and altered movement patterns up to 9 months after ACL surgery, which impair safe return to sport.[44]

Further testing has also noted up to a 43% deficit in knee joint power absorption and a 6% decrease in extensor moment with a single-leg hop test 7 months after surgery.[45] This decrease in knee loading and accommodating force at the knee is a major concern, as knee flexion control contributes between 40% and 55% of the power absorption of the lower body with running.[46,47] Rates of force development have also been studied and it was found out that the rates of activation of the quadriceps, hamstrings, and gluteal muscles during running and jumping were significantly slower than those in the unaffected leg.[48]

Patients status post ACLR have also been shown to have thinner cartilage around the femoral condyles of their injured leg compared with their uninjured side.[49] This decreased cartilage thickness coincides with decreased quadriceps function as well as an increased risk of developing early osteoarthritis (OA) in the surgically repaired knee. The risk of early onset of OA is significantly increased when meniscal injury accompanies the original ACL tear.

One additional aspect to be considered is kinesiophobia or fear of movement, which should be addressed as part of the psychologic aspects of returning to sports. Patients who have increased apprehension and fear of reinjuring their surgically repaired knee tend to have stiffer jumping and landing mechanics and as a result put themselves at a greater risk of reinjury.[50]

With even the best rehabilitation program and a wide array of functional testing, it is inevitable that there will be some strength and proprioceptive deficits status post ACLR and it is up to the rehabilitation professional to minimize these deficits as much as possible. While an athletic competition cannot truly be replicated in the clinical setting, a thorough rehabilitation program should include multiple variables such as different playing surfaces, different speeds of movement for both acceleration and deceleration movements, and incorporation of obstacles to simulate real-life situations for a given athlete. The more an athlete is challenged in the clinic, the more the athlete will be physically and mentally prepared to handle any challenges that they may face on the field of play.

REFERENCES

1. Sackett DL. Evidence based medicine: what it is and what it isn't. *BMJ.* 1996;312:71.
2. Sepulveda F, Sanchez L, Amy E, Micheo W. Anterior cruciate ligament injury: return to play, function, and long-term considerations. *Curr Sports Med Rep.* 2017;16(3):172–178.
3. Barber-Westin SD, Noyes FR, Tutalo Smith S, Campbell TM. Reducing the risk of noncontact anterior cruciate ligament injuries in female athletes. *Phys Sports Med.* 2009;37(3):49–61.
4. Barber-Westin SD, Noyes FR. Factors used to determine return to unrestricted sports activities after anterior cruciate ligament reconstruction. *J Arthr Relat Surg.* 2011;27(12):1697–1705.
5. Hewett TE, Lindenfeld TN, Riccobene JV, Noyes FR. The effect of neuromuscular training on the incidence of knee injury in female athletes. *Am J Sports Med.* 1996;27(6):699–706.
6. Pfeiffer TR, Kanakamedala AC, Herbst E, et al. Female sex is associated with greater rotatory knee laxity in collegiate athletes. *Knee Surg Sports Traumatol Arthrosc.* August 19, 2017. https://doi.org/10.10007/s00167-017-4684-6. (Epub ahead of print).
7. Wright, et al. Systematic review of ACL reconstruction rehabilitation Part 1. *J Knee Surg.* 2008.
8. Kruse LM, Gray B, Wright RW. Rehabilitation after anterior cruciate ligament reconstruction. A systematic review. *J Bone Joint Surg Am.* 2012;94:1737–1748.
9. Hauger AV, Reiman MP, Bjordal JM, Sheets C, Ledbetter L, Goode AP. Neuromuscular electrical stimulation is effective in strengthening the quadriceps muscle after anterior cruciate ligament surgery. *Knee Surg Sports Traumatol Arthrosc.* August 17, 2017. https://doi.org/10.1007/s00167-017-4669-5. (Epub ahead of print).
10. Wicke J, Gainey K, Figueroa M. A comparison of self-administered proprioceptive neuromuscular facilitation to static stretching on range of motion and flexibility. *J Strength Cond Res.* 2014;28(1):169–172.
11. Escamilla RF, Fleisig GS, Zheng N, Barrentine SW, Wilk KE, Andrews JR. Biomechanics of the knee during closed kinetic chain and open kinetic chain exercises. *Med Sci Sports Exerc.* 1998;30(4):556–569.
12. Stavrinou ML, Della Penna S, Pizzella V, et al. Temporal dynamics of plastic changes in human primary somatosensory cortex after finger webbing. *Cereb Cortex.* 2007;17:2134–2142.
13. Cinar-Medeni O, Baltaci G, Bayramlar K, Yanmis I. Core stability, knee muscle strength, and anterior translation are correlated with postural stability in anterior cruciate ligament-reconstructed patients. *Am J Phys Med Rehabil.* 2015;94(4):280–287.
14. Velazquez-Saornil J, Ruiz-Ruiz B, Rodriguez-Sanz D, et al. Efficacy of quadriceps vastus medialis dry needling in a rehabilitation protocol after surgical reconstruction of complete anterior cruciate ligament rupture. *Medicine.* 2017;96(17):e6726.
15. Kraeutler MJ, Wolsky RM, Vidal AF, Bravman JT. Anatomy and biomechanics of the native and reconstructed Wanterior cruciate ligament: surgical implications. *J Bone Joint Surg.* 2017;99:438–445.
16. Kaeding CC, Pedroza AD, Reinke EK, et al. Risk factors of subsequent ACL injury in either knee after ACL reconstruction: prospective analysis of 2488 primary ACL reconstructions from the MOON cohort. *Am J Sports Med.* 2015;43(7):1583–1590.
17. Barrett GR, Luber K, Replogle WH, Manley JL. Allograft anterior cruciate ligament reconstruction in the young, active patient: tegner activity level and failure rate. *Arthroscopy.* 2010;26(12):1593–1601.
18. Kyritsis P, Bahr R, Landreau P, et al. Likelihood of ACL graft rupture: not meeting six clinical discharge criteria before return to sport is associated with a four times greater risk of rupture. *Br J Sports Med.* 2016;50(15):946–951.
19. Baumgart C, et al. Do ground reaction forces during unilateral and bilateral movements exhibit compensation strategies following ACL reconstruction? *Knee Surg Sports Traumatol Arthrosc.* 2017. (in press) https://doi.org/10.1007/s00167015-3623-7.
20. Wojtys EM, Huston LJ, Schock HJ, et al. Gender differences in muscular protection of the knee in torsion in size-matched athletes. *J Bone Joint Surg.* 2003:782–795.
21. Schoenfeld BJ. Potential mechanisms for a role of metabolic stress in hypertrophic adaptations to resistance training. *Sports Med.* 2013;43(3):179–194.
22. Takarada Y, Takazawa H, Sato Y, Takebayashi S, Ishii N. Effects of resistance exercise combined with moderate vascular occlusion on muscular function in humans. *J Appl Physiol.* 2000;88:2097–2106.
23. Wilson JM, Lowery RP, Joy JM, Loenneke JP, Naimo MA. Practical blood flow restriction raining increases acute determinants of hypertrophy without increasing indices of muscle damage. *J Strength Cond Res.* 2013;27(11):3068–3075.
24. Poton R, Polito MD. Hemodynamic response to resistance exercise with and without blood flow restriction in healthy subjects. *Clin Physiol Funct Imaging.* 2014. https://doi.org/10.1111/cpf.12218.
25. Laurentino GC, Ugrinowitsch C, Roschel H, et al. Strength training with blood flow restriction diminishes myostatin gene expression. *Med Sci Sports Exerc.* 2012;44(3):406–412.
26. Loenneke JP, Wilson JM, Marin PJ, et al. Low intensity blood flow restriction training: a meta-analysis. *Eur J Sport Sci.* 2012;112(5):1849–1859.
27. Giugliano DN, Solomon JL. ACL tears in female athletes. *Phys Med Rehab Clin North Am.* 2007;18(3):417–438.
28. Barber-Westin SD, Noyes FR. Objective criteria for return to athletics after anterior cruciate ligament reconstruction and subsequent reinjury rates: a systematic review. *Phys Sports Med.* 2011;39(3):100–110.
29. MacWilliams BA, Wilson DR, DesJardins JD, et al. Hamstrings co-contraction reduces internal rotation, anterior translation, and anterior cruciate ligament load in weight-bearing flexion. *J Orthop Res.* 1999;17(6):817–822.
30. Palmeiri-Smith RM, Thomas AC, Wojtys EM. Maximizing quadriceps strength after ACL reconstruction. *Clin Sports Med.* 2008;27(3):405–424.

31. Solomonow M, Baratta R, Zhou BH, et al. The synergistic action of the anterior cruciate ligament and thigh muscles in maintaining joint stability. *Am J Sports Med.* 1987;15(3):207–213.

32. Kline PW, Johnson DL, Ireland ML, Noehren B. Clinical predictors of knee mechanics and return to sport after ACL reconstruction. *Med Sci Sports Exerc.* 2016;48(5):790–795.

33. Noyes FR, Barber SD, Mangine RE. Abnormal lower limb symmetry determined by function hop tests after anterior cruciate ligament rupture. *Am J Sports Med.* 1991;19:513–518.

34. Reid A, Birmingham TB, Stratford PW, Alcock GK, Giffin JR. Hop testing provides a reliable and valid outcome measure during rehabilitation after anterior cruciate ligament reconstruction. *Phys Ther.* 2007;87(3):337–348.

35. Ardern CL, Webster KE, Taylor NF, Feller JA. Return to sport following anterior cruciate ligament reconstruction surgery: a systematic review and meta-analysis of the state of play. *Br J Sports Med.* 2011;45:596–606.

36. Shah VM, Andrews JR, Fleisig GS, McMichael CS, Lemark LJ. Return to play after anterior cruciate ligament reconstruction in national football league athletes. *Am J Sports Med.* 2010;38:2233–2239.

37. Busfield BT, Kharrazi FD, Starkey C, Lombardo SJ, Seegmiller J. Performance outcomes of anterior cruciate ligament reconstruction in the national basketball association. *Arthroscopy.* 2009;25:825–830.

38. Fabricant PD, Chin CS, Conte S, et al. Return to play after anterior cruciate ligament reconstruction in major league baseball athletes. *J Arthrosc Rel Surg.* 2015;31(5):896–900.

39. Dekker TJ, Godin JA, Dale KM, et al. Return to sport after pediatric anterior cruciate ligament reconstruction and its effect on subsequent anterior cruciate ligament injury. *J Bone Joint Surg.* 2017;99(11):897–904.

40. Chmielewski TL. Asymmetrical lower extremity loading after ACL reconstruction: more than meets the eye. *J Ortho Sports Phys Ther.* 2011:374–376.

41. Ernst GP, et al. Lower extremity compensations following anterior cruciate ligament reconstruction. *Phys Ther.* 2000;80:251–260.

42. Fukunaga T, McHugh MP, Johnson CD, Nicholas SJ. *To what Extent Is Weakness after ACL Reconstruction Due to Central Inhibition versus Muscle Atrophy? a Magnetic Stimulation Study.* New York, NY: Northwell Health Lenox Hill Hospital; 2017.

43. Boyle MJ, Butler RJ, Queen RM. Functional movement competency and dynamic balance after anterior cruciate ligament reconstruction in adolescent patients. *J Pediatr Orthop.* 2016;36:36–41.

44. Orishimo KF, et al. Adaptations in single leg hop biomechanics following anterior cruciate ligament reconstruction. *Knee Surg Sports Traumatol Arthrosc.* 2010;18:1587–1593.

45. Scache AG, et al. Modulation of work and power by the human lower-limb joints with increasing steady-state locomotion speed. *J Exp Biol.* 2015;218:2472–2481.

46. Pratt KA, Sigward SM. Knee loading deficits during dynamic tasks in individuals following anterior cruciate ligament reconstruction. *J Orthop Sports Phys Ther.* 2017;47(6):411–419.

47. Cobian DG, Knurr KA, Stiffler MR, et al. Reduced rates of quadriceps activation during running and jumping in collegiate athletes post-ACL reconstruction. *Med Sci Sports Exerc.* 2017;49(5 suppl 1):S374.

48. Pamukoff DN, Montgomery MM, Moffit TJ, Vakula MN. Quadriceps function and knee joint ultrasonography following ACL reconstruction. *Med Sci Sports Exerc.* 2017. https://doi.org/10.1249/MSS.0000000000001437. (epub ahead of print).

49. Trigsted SM, Post E, Schaefer D, et al. The effect of fear of reinjury on biomechanics during a jump landing following ACL reconstruction. *Med Sci Sports Exerc.* 2017;49(5 suppl 1):S374.

ADDITIONAL REFERENCES

1. Foster JB. ACLR aftershocks: deficits linger after return to sports. *Low Extrem Rev.* 2017;9(6):13–14.

2. Hewett TE, Stroupe AL, Nance TA, Noyes FR. Plyometric training in female athletes. *Am J Sports Med.* 1996;24(6):765–773.

3. Hewett TE. Prediction of future injury in sport: primary and secondary anterior cruciate ligament injury risk and return to sport as a model. *J Orthop Sports Phys Ther.* 2017;47(4):228–231.

4. Jordan MJ, Aagaard P, Herzog W. Rapid hamstrings/quadriceps strength in ACL-reconstructed elite alpine ski racers. *Med Sci Sports Exerc.* 2015;47(1):109–119.

5. Kubo K, Komuro T, Ishiguro N, et al. Effects of low-load resistance training with vascular occlusion on the mechanical properties of muscle and tendon. *J Appl Biomech.* 2006;22(2):112–119.

6. Loenneke JP, Balapur A, Thrower AD, Barnes JT, Pujol TJ. Blood flow restriction reduces time to muscular failure. *Eur J Sport Sci.* 2012:238–243.

7. Ohta H, et al. Low-load resistance muscular training with moderate restriction of blood flow after anterior cruciate ligament reconstruction. *Acta Orthop.* 2003;74(1):62–68.

8. Ransdell LB, Murray T. Functional movement screening: an important tool for female athletes. *Strength Cond J.* 1996;38(2):40–48.

9. Takarada Y, Nakamura Y, Aruga S, Onda T, Miyazaki S, Ishii N. Rapid increase in plasma growth hormone after low-intensity resistance exercise with vascular occlusion. *J Appl Physiol 1985.* 2000;88:61–65.

10. Wojtys EM, Ashton-Miller JA, Huston LJ. A gender-related difference in the contribution of the knee musculature to sagittal-plane shear stiffness in subjects with similar knee laxity. *J Bone Joint Surg.* 2002;84-A(1):10–16.

11. Xergia SA, Pappas E, Zampeli F. Asymmetries in functional hop tests, lower extremity kinematics, and isokinetic strength persist 6 to 9 months following anterior cruciate ligament reconstruction. *JOSPT.* 2013;43(3):154–162.

CHAPTER 10

The Future: Orthobiologics and Anterior Cruciate Ligament Injury

ELEONOR SVANTESSON, MD, PHD • MARCIN KOWALCZUK, MD •
AJAY KANAKAMEDALA, MD • LEE SASALA, MD • VOLKER MUSAHL, MD

INTRODUCTION

The anterior cruciate ligament (ACL) rarely heals spontaneously after rupture,[1-5] and numerous studies have attempted to elucidate the underlying causes of the ACL's poor healing potential. It was initially believed that many of the ACL's barriers to healing were intrinsic to the ACL, such as a limited blood supply[6-8] and slower migration and proliferation of fibroblasts within the ACL.[9,10] There is growing evidence, however, that the main barriers to ACL healing may not be an intrinsic lack of healing potential but extrinsic factors that ultimately disturb a crucial step in the ligament healing process, the formation of a fibrin clot.[11-13] Intra-articular synovial fluid contains several factors, including enzymes and proinflammatory cytokines, whose concentrations increase after ACL rupture.[14-17] These factors may lead to impaired fibrin clot formation, inadequate wound site filling, and, ultimately, impaired ACL healing.[11,18,19] Moreover, unlike the medial collateral ligament, which has been shown to have a robust healing response to injury,[20,21] the ACL does not have a surrounding soft tissue envelope and is encased only by a thin layer of synovium. This layer is typically disrupted during ACL injuries, leaving the ACL without a stable scaffold for a fibrin clot to form.[13]

While primary repair of the ACL may work in selected patients,[22,23] multiple studies have reported discouraging results with rates of subjective instability as high as 90% and reoperation in up to two-thirds of patients.[24-26] Nevertheless, the ACL is capable of exhibiting a proliferative response to rupture[27-29] and even spontaneous healing.[30] This has led to an interest in the potential uses of biological techniques in the augmentation of both primary ACL healing and direct repair, which has multiple potential benefits, including the preservation of native ACL physiology, biomechanics, and proprioception.[31,32]

The poor outcomes associated with primary repair have led to a shift toward reconstruction of the ACL, which is now the gold standard for operative treatment.

Despite numerous advances in technique, ACL reconstruction (ACLR) does continue to have limitations, including donor site morbidity,[33] increased risk of developing osteoarthritis,[34,35] as well as altered biomechanics and gait dynamics.[36-40] Graft failure after ACLR is another notable complication that typically tends to occur at the tendon-to-bone or graft-to-bone interface.[41-43]

Given the advances in biological techniques, there is now an increased interest in the use of biologics to augment primary healing, direct repair, and reconstruction of the ACL. For example, stem cells could be utilized to modify the intra-articular environment to promote both native ACL and graft-to-bone healing and biological scaffolds could provide a stable framework to facilitate fibrin clot formation. This chapter focuses on the use of growth factors, stem cell scaffolds, and platelet-rich plasma (PRP) in the biological augmentation of primary healing, repair, and reconstruction of the ACL.

GROWTH FACTORS

Numerous growth factors have been suggested to influence the healing process of the ACL. Growth factors aid in ACL repair by improving the fibroblast healing environment.[44] Growth factors increase cell proliferation, increase extracellular matrix deposition, promote vascularization, and improve the biomechanical properties of the tissue. This ultimately leads to improved graft incorporation, strength, and remodeling.[45] Fibroblast growth factor (FGF), transforming growth factor (TGF), and epidermal growth factor have been studied most extensively in the literature in various animal in vitro and a few in vivo models.[44-49] But to date, there have been no human studies demonstrating any benefit to ACL repair or ACLR. More work is needed in the future to determine if these promising laboratory findings will become beneficial clinically. The study of growth factors remains important because it provides insight into the mechanism of action of other orthobiologics such as, stem cells and PRP.

ACL Injuries in Female Athletes. https://doi.org/10.1016/B978-0-323-54839-7.00010-5

BIOLOGICAL AGENTS TO FACILITATE BONE TUNNEL HEALING

The incorporation of graft material into the tibial and femoral tunnels is critical for successful ACLR. For this to occur, inflammatory cells and bone marrow–derived stem cells must migrate to the interface between the graft and bone.[5] The bone-soft tissue graft interface is the weakest point of the reconstruction during the early postoperative period.[50] Biological adjuncts that accelerate the process of graft healing and maturation could theoretically allow earlier and more aggressive rehabilitation, with the potential for earlier return to full activity.[5,51]

The native ACL insertion has a fibrocartilage tissue that connects to the deeper layer of bone.[51] This includes four distinct tissues: tendon, fibrocartilage, mineralized fibrocartilage, and bone. This complex architecture is not recreated during either ACLR or healing.[52] Soft tissue graft-to-bone healing occurs more slowly than bone-to-bone healing, such as that occurring in bone-patella-bone grafts, because of the avascularity of the fibrocartilage zone and bone loss at the tunnel.[53] Moreover, the normal healing process can result in a fibrous scar-like tissue at the tendon-bone interface.[53,54] This fibrous layer is weak and at risk for failure.[55]

For the abovementioned reasons, particular attention has been focused on the methods of accelerating graft-bone tunnel healing with the use of orthobiologics, namely, stem cells and PRP. For example, in an animal study an engineered CD34+ cell sheet was wrapped around a tendon graft, leading to improved bone-tendon healing and graft formation.[56] Building upon this body of work, in a subsequent study, bone morphogenetic protein (BMP) 2 was also added to the grafts wrapped in CD34+ stem cell sheet.[57] The addition of BMP to the stem cells significantly increased the graft-bone incorporation and the biomechanical strength as measured by tensile load to failure.[57] Multiple studies have shown positive results for PRP on the proliferation of osteoblasts and tenocytes in graft-bone healing.[50,58] PRP has also been shown to promote vascularization and reinnervation of the graft, which was proposed to explain the promotion of graft maturation by PRP.[59] Although there has been some promising bench studies and animal models using PRP, no study has shown a statistically significant difference in clinical outcome, tunnel widening, or graft incorporation.[60]

Stem Cells

One major impediment to ACL healing involves the intra-articular environment of the knee, which is believed to contain factors that disturb fibrin clot formation, leading to impaired ACL healing.[11,18,19] In searching for ways to modify the intra-articular environment to optimize the ACL's healing potential, researchers have identified stem cells as a possible solution. Stem cells are pluripotent cells with the capacity to replicate indefinitely and the ability to differentiate into several cell types.[61,62] Although various types of stem cells have been studied for their use in ACL healing, including vascular stem cells[63] and ACL-derived stem cells,[56,64,65] the mesenchymal stem cells (MSCs) are probably the most studied for their potential uses in primary ACL healing and ACLR.[12,61,62,66–68]

MSCs are nonhematopoietic stromal cells that have the ability to differentiate into chondrocytes, osteoblasts, fibroblasts, and adipocytes, i.e., the constituents of mesenchymal tissues, such as ligaments, bone, and cartilage.[61,62,66,69] They can be acquired from various sources including bone marrow, adipose, muscle, and even perivascular tissues.[61,62,67,69] There is evidence that MSCs migrate out of the damaged ACL and increase in concentration in the synovial fluid after ACL injury.[70,71] There are several animal studies that suggest that MSCs may improve graft-to-bone healing.[72–76] It was initially thought that their primary mechanism of action was related to their mobilization into injured tissues and subsequent differentiation and proliferation to fabricate new tissues.[61,66,67] An equally important role may, however, be played by both their immunomodulatory effects, which suppress inflammatory reactions that impair healing, and their secretory effects, including the production and secretion of important factors such as TGF-β1.[66,67,77–79] For their effects on tissue fabrication and healing, MSCs have been proposed in the biological augmentation of both primary ACL healing and ACLR.

Use of mesenchymal stem cells in animals

To determine whether MSCs could mobilize into injured tissues in rats' knees, one study surgically injured the ACL, medial meniscus, and articular cartilage and performed intra-articular injections of green fluorescent protein-positive MSCs into the knees of eight rats. This study demonstrated signs of MSC mobilization into the ACL of all eight knees and into the medial meniscus and articular cartilage of six knees, suggesting that intra-articular injection may serve as an adequate delivery method for biological augmentation of ACL healing with MSCs.

Building upon this work, another study performed intra-articular injections of MSCs into rat knees with partially transected ACL and evaluated for histologic signs of healing and conducted biomechanical testing to compare the tensile strengths of the ACL in each group.[80] It was found that in the MSC group, there were greater histologic scores and visibly healed tissue in the transected area, as well as a higher ultimate failure load of the femur-ACL-tibia complex, suggesting that intra-articular injection of MSCs led to significantly improved ACL healing when compared with the control group.

In a similar rat study, intra-articular injections of bone marrow stem cells (BMSCs), MSCs, and saline were performed 1 week after partial ACL transection.[77] It was found that the tensile strength of the femur-ACL-tibia complexes in both the BMC and MSC groups was significantly greater than that of the control group at the 2- and 4-week time points. Significantly greater levels of TGF-β1 in the knee joint fluid and greater amounts of tenocytes and collagen fibers were also found at the 4-week time point.[70,71,77,80,81]

One noteworthy limitation to these animal studies is that there may be significant discrepancies between the intra-articular environment of surgically transected ACLs and that of the traumatically injured ACLs that are not captured by these models. The difficulty in developing such a model is exemplified by the fact that all the animal studies cited here that have examined ACL injury have performed some form of surgical transection of the ACL to mimic ACL injury. Future efforts will be valuable in creating a more realistic model of ACL injury in animals.

Use of mesenchymal stem cells in humans

In a prospective case series of 10 patients with grade I–III ACL injury (grade III in five patients) and less than 1 cm of retraction, PRP and bone marrow concentrate (BMC) were injected into the remaining ACL tissue under fluoroscopic control.[82] Prior to this injection, patients were injected with a hypertonic dextrose solution, which the authors suggested would establish a prompt inflammatory response and stimulate healing and cell proliferation.[83,84] At 3 months' follow-up, improved ligamentization on MRI and improved functional scores were found in seven patients. No objective measurements of knee stability were performed.

Although there was no control group, it was suggested that the results were due to the treatment protocol, and not natural healing, as grade II and III ACL injuries typically do not heal spontaneously. While this study did not look at the effects of MSCs exclusively, it was postulated that, given the numerous studies showing the limited effect of PRP on ACL healing, this study would mostly be evaluating the effects of the MSCs and hematopoietic stem cells present in the BMC.

In a prospective study, 43 patients undergoing ACLR were randomized to undergo either a typical ACLR or an ACLR with injections of stem cells both into the femoral end of the graft and in the tunnel around the graft.[85] No difference was found in graft-to-bone healing based on MRI evaluation, and it was concluded that the use of adult noncultivated BMSCs does not appear to accelerate graft-to-bone healing after ACLR. Given that the concentration of stem cells in the concentrate was not measured prior to injection, the observed results might have been due to subtherapeutic concentrations of MSCs in the BMSC concentrates.

In summary, animal studies[77,80,81] have provided promising results for the beneficial effect of intra-articular injections of MSCs to augment both primary ACL healing and ACLR. In partial ACL tears and in the setting of ACLR, based on the evidence from the two human studies presented,[82,85] there is currently insufficient data to support or reject the use of MSCs in ACLR. Given the small number of human studies on the use of MSCs for ACL repair and ACLR, further studies will be particularly valuable in this area. While several studies have investigated the use of intra-articular injections as a vehicle of delivery for MSCs, there continues to be exploration into other methods of delivering MSCs, such as cell sheets[56] or with other biologics such as scaffolds.[86–89]

Scaffolds for Biological Augmentation

Because of the tensile properties of the ACL and absence of blood clot formation following ACL rupture, the torn ends of the ACL retract significantly from each other, impeding natural healing.[22,90] In an effort to facilitate healing, a scaffold represents a potential means to bridge the ends of the ruptured ACL and create a favorable environment for migrating and proliferating cells. Moreover, a scaffold can act as a potential source of cytokines and growth factors beneficial for ACL healing, including growth hormone, FGF, and TGF-β.[91–94] The ideal structural scaffold should not only mimic the shape and kinematic properties of the native ACL but also be biodegradable with a degradation profile that permits sufficient time for neotissue formation and regeneration.[95–97]

As the ACL consists of approximately 90% type I collagen, collagen-based scaffolds have been subject to extensive investigation.[95,98] Scaffolds consisting of aligned type I collagen from porcine small intestinal submucosa (SIS) have shown promising results in animal studies of ligament repair.[99] When evaluating the histologic characteristics of transected goat ACLs treated with suture and an SIS scaffold, it was shown that the fibers of the ACL were denser and more compactly arranged after augmentation with SIS scaffold when compared with suture repair alone.[100] In a similar study, an SIS scaffold was combined with SIS hydrogel to repair the ACL in skeletally mature goats. Compared with animals treated with suture alone, the SIS-treated group showed superior neotissue formation, 4.5 times increased cross-sectional area of the ACL, and a significantly greater stiffness of the femur-ACL-tibia complexes after 12 weeks. Furthermore, the cross-sectional area of the ACL was comparable to that of the sham-operated contralateral hind limb, which was visualized by opening the joint without transecting the ACL.[101]

Although the use of collagen-based scaffolds has been proposed to significantly improve primary ACL repair, the technique may be insufficient alone and may require supplementation with other bioactive materials.[22,102] In addition to supplementation with hydrogel, supplementing collagen scaffolds with autologous platelets has been shown beneficial to promote ACL healing. A large amount of fibrin-degrading proteases circulate in the synovial fluid following ACL rupture. When a fibrin clot is used for delivery of platelets, it may consequently be dissolved by these proteases, ultimately leading to treatment failure.[22] However, the combination of a fibrin and a collagen scaffold has been reported to be more resistant to degradation,[18] and the platelets may consequently function at the wound site for a longer period. The addition of collagen is also advantageous because it allows for a prolonged release period of platelet-associated factors compared with physiologic release.[103] Primary repair in porcine models using a suture stent and a collagen scaffold soaked with whole blood to deliver platelets has been reported to be equivalent to ACLR in terms of biomechanical characteristics at 3, 6, and 12 months.[104–106] Furthermore, this technique led to improved prevention of the development of cartilage lesions at 12 months when compared with both untreated ACL transection and ACLR.[106]

However, a notable disadvantage of collagen scaffolds is that their mechanical strength decreases over time owing to the fast resorption of the material. Furthermore, concerns over immunologic reactions against bovine collagen[95,107] and leakage of chemical cross-linking agents have been raised.[95] As a result, an interest in silk-based scaffolds has evolved. Silk is biocompatible, has a long turnover time, and offers tensile properties similar to those of the native ACL.[96,108,109] The remarkable strength of silk fibrin is especially beneficial during the period of neotissue formation when processes such as collagen alignment and vascularization are facilitated by the stability provided by the silk structure.[96] Large animal studies have evaluated this scaffold technique and provided encouraging results.[88,110] Interestingly, a hybrid scaffold consisting of both collagen and silk was developed in an attempt to take advantage of the degradation profile of collagen, while enhancing the strength by using the silk fibers.[111] Scaffolds consisting of ≥25% silk showed greater tensile strength than the native ACL. However, given the slow resorption rate of silk, a reduction in its volume and further efforts to find materials with a more favorable degradation profile are needed.[111]

The majority of studies of scaffolds for ACL repair have been conducted in animal models. However, Murray et al.,[112] reported on the use of a scaffold technique for primary ACL repair in humans. The bridge-enhanced ACL repair (BEAR) technique is built on two fundamentals. First, biological enhancement of the healing is facilitated by incorporation of a bioactive scaffold loaded with autologous whole blood. Second, mechanical stabilization of the knee is provided by suture repair of the ACL. The BEAR scaffold is composed of extracellular matrix proteins and includes collagen obtained from bovine tissue. It has a length of 45 mm and a diameter of 22 mm and is able to absorb five times its weight in fluid.[112] Prior preclinical studies have showed that the scaffold is resorbed by 95% within 6 weeks and fully resorbed at 8 weeks.[113]

In order to be considered for the BEAR procedure, patients must have sustained an ACL injury within 1 month from examination and have tibial attachment stumps of the ACL of at least 50% of its original length on preoperative MRI.[112] In the study, 10 patients underwent the BEAR procedure and another 10 patients underwent ACLR with hamstring tendon autograft. Both groups had a mean age of 24 years. At 3 months' follow-up, the two groups were comparable on clinical examination in terms of regained stability, knee range of motion, hip abduction, and International Knee Documentation Committee (IKDC) score. On Lachman examination according to the IKDC, a grade A result was found in 8 of the 10 patients in the BEAR group, implicating a firm endpoint and −1 to 2-mm side-to-side difference compared with the contralateral leg. Furthermore, there was no difference in return to school/work, the duration of the use of crutches, or the thigh circumference. The BEAR scaffold was well tolerated by the intra-articular milieu and did not cause any deep infections or serious inflammatory reactions. The only significant difference between the groups was seen in hamstring strength, where the BEAR group was favored in terms of a higher limb symmetry ratio than the group who underwent ACLR. The authors stressed that one of the main advantages of the BEAR scaffold is that exact reapproximation of the torn

ACL is not required because the scaffold fills the gap between the ends, which is further enhanced by the addition of autologous blood to the scaffold. Other repair techniques often need reapproximation under compression, which requires that a significant length of the tibial stump must remain. This is seldom seen in ACL tears and therefore limits the applicability of such repair techniques. Although this study on bioactive scaffolds, the first in humans, showed encouraging results, there is still need for further comprehensive research on primary ACL repair enhanced by using scaffolds before it may be fully implemented in the clinical setting.

Platelet-Rich Plasma

Among the various orthobiologics studied for use in ACL injuries, PRP has been the most extensively investigated. Upon activation, platelets release various growth factors including platelet-derived growth factor, vascular endothelial growth factor, FGF, and TGF-β1; these factors modulate tissue healing through the inflammatory and remodeling phases.[114,115] Laboratory data suggests that high local concentration of these growth factors leads to an enhanced chemotactic effect, which increases type I collagen production.[116]

PRP is prepared from a sample of autologous anticoagulated blood that has been centrifuged or filtered to obtain a sample high in platelets and the noncellular components of plasma, including growth factors.[114] The desired concentration of platelets/growth factors, the volume of the final preparation, the inclusion of leukocytes into the preparation, and the use of activating agents and delivery method vary widely in the literature, making the interpretation of study data regarding clinical efficacy difficult.[115,117] Furthermore, the exact concentration of platelets is dependent not only on the system used for preparation but also on the patient's baseline laboratory values.

In the setting of ACL injury, PRP has been used both to augment traditional ACLR and to aid in the healing or repair of partial tears. When used to augment traditional ACLR, four potential roles of PRP have been investigated. These include the enlargement of ACL boney tunnels, ACL graft-bone interface integration, ACL graft maturation, and overall clinical results, which include return to sport.

In a randomized controlled trial (RCT) investigating femoral tunnel widening, 51 patients were evaluated after receiving PRP injection directly into the tunnel at the time of ACLR.[118] Decreased tunnel widening was observed at the midsubstance of the tunnel, but no difference was observed at the proximal or distal tunnel

apertures at 12 months. Clinical results were equivalent between groups.

Several additional RCTs have further investigated the effect of PRP on tunnel widening. Each of these studies reported no effect, and given the short-term follow-up and the equivalent clinical results observed in the study described earlier, the use of PRP to reduce tunnel enlargement after ACLR with bone-tendon-bone (BTB) autograft or soft tissue grafts cannot be recommended.[118–125]

The effect of PRP on ACL soft tissue graft and tunnel bone interface integration has also been investigated in several RCTs, with the majority showing no effect.[121,124,126–128] PRP has been injected under direct visualization into the femoral or tibial tunnels, injected into the substance of the graft, or sewn into the graft between the limbs of semitendinosus/gracilis graft during preparation in an attempt to target delivery. Vogrin et al.[129] at 4–6 weeks after ACLR reported increased vascularization at the osteoligamentous interface in patients who received PRP intraoperatively when compared with controls. No evidence of neovascularization of the intra-articular portion of the graft was however reported. In a separate RCT, the effect of PRP on tunnel cortical bone deposition was evaluated in 50 patients using MRI. Those who received PRP were found to have a significantly greater proportion (67.1% vs. 53.5%) of sclerotic bone encircling the treated bone tunnels at 6 months after surgery.[130] Patient-reported outcomes were not reported.

Mixed results have been noted in RCTs evaluating the effect of PRP on graft maturation after ACLR. In a study of 98 patients, improved graft maturity was observed by MRI at 4 and 6 months, but by 12 months after operation, the results were equal to the control group.[131] All patients underwent ACLR with BTB autograft and had 8 mL of PRP injected into the intra-articular space after wound closure. Additional trials have confirmed these results by using hamstring autograft for ACLR.[121,132,133] The evidence for improved graft maturation is, however, not uniform, with several studies showing no effect.[127,129] Although the majority of the evidence in the literature does point to accelerated and improved graft maturity at 6 months after operation, the clinical significance of this remains unclear. Furthermore, surgeons should factor in the additional cost, given the graft maturity is likely equivalent by 12 months in patients treated with and without PRP.[60]

Ultimately, the efficacy of PRP can be evaluated by examining clinical outcomes. Prospective data from an unblinded consecutive case series of patients who underwent ACLR with or without PRP augmentation revealed no difference in objective IKDC or Rolimeter measurements but did note IKDC subjective scores to be significantly higher (78±5.3 vs. 65.1±9.8) in the PRP group at 24 months after operation.[126] In an RCT involving 45 patients who underwent ACLR with double-looped semitendinosus and gracilis autograft, it was reported that application of a PRP (leukocyte rich) gel to the tunnels and graft resulted in a significant decrease in KT-2000 measurements (6.7±2.1 mm vs. 4.7±1.9 mm) at 6 months.[129] Three systematic reviews of literature have confirmed that, to date, no other studies have reported a statistically significant or minimal clinically important difference in patient-reported outcomes of augmentation of ACLR with PRP.[117,120,122] Given the current evidence, routine use of PRP in the setting of ACLR cannot be recommended.

The use of PRP has also been investigated in the treatment of partial ACL tears and in cases of attempted ACL repair.[134] In a case series of 19 high-level European footballers with arthroscopically confirmed isolated tears of the anteromedial bundle of the ACL and resultant instability treated with a 4-mL injection of PRP into the intact bundle, successful return to play was observed in all but one patient.[135] All but three patients returned to play at their previous level with no evidence of instability on clinical examination and good ligamentization of the remaining bundle was observed on MRI at 1 year after injury.

Historically, the outcomes of ACL repair have been poor. Improved knowledge and surgical techniques have, however, revived interest in this procedure, given the potential benefits in knee kinematics and patient proprioception when compared with ACLR. In a case series, suture repair of partial ACL tears was coupled with marrow stimulation and injection of PRP.[136] At 5 years' follow-up, 78% of the 58 treated patients were reported to be back to athletic activities and side-to-side differences in anteroposterior translation were 1.4±0.8 mm compared with 4.1±1.6 mm preoperatively. No control group or reconstruction group was available for comparison.

PRP has been one of the most extensively studied orthobiological agents in patients with ACL injuries. To date, however, the available evidence does not support routine use of PRP in the treating ACL injury.[117,120,122,134] As techniques such as the use of bioscaffolds in conjunction with PRP continue to evolve, PRP continues to represent an important area of study. Large, well-designed, high-quality clinical trials with extended follow-up using standardized PRP preparations will be imperative in confirming clinical efficacy.[115]

CONCLUSION

Advances in orthobiological techniques have led to increased interest in augmentation of ACL healing, primary repair, and reconstruction. To date, most evidence is based on animal studies, which have shown promising results such as increased cell proliferation, increased vascularization, and improved graft maturity. There is paucity of human studies and the results of human investigations are inconclusive. Among the various orthobiologics studied for use in human ACL injuries, PRP has been extensively investigated. However, the clinically important impact of augmentation with PRP alone is questionable. A plausible future approach is to utilize a combination of biological agents and tissue engineering approaches to achieve a synergistic function of orthobiologics. The advancement of scaffolds and orthobiologics in the human population will hopefully provide valuable insights into further developing the approaches for the biological augmentation of ACL repair.

REFERENCES

1. Woo SL, Debski RE, Withrow JD, Janaushek MA. Biomechanics of knee ligaments. *Am J Sports Med.* 1999;27(4):533–543.
2. Woo SL-Y, Vogrin TM, Abramowitch SD. Healing and repair of ligament injuries in the knee. *J Am Acad Orthop Surg.* 2000;8(6):364–372.
3. Wasmaier J, Kubik-Huch R, Pfirrmann C, Grehn H, Bieg C, Eid K. Proximal anterior cruciate ligament tears: the healing response technique versus conservative treatment. *J Knee Surg.* 2013;26(04):263–272.
4. Johnson RJ, Beynnon BD, Nichols CE, Renstrom P. The treatment of injuries of the anterior cruciate ligament. *JBJS.* 1992;74(1):140–151.
5. Vavken P, Murray MM. The potential for primary repair of the ACL. *Sports Med Arthrosc Rev.* 2011;19(1):44.
6. Alm A, Strömberg B. Vascular anatomy of the patellar and cruciate ligaments. A microangiographic and histologic investigation in the dog. *Acta Chirurgica Scand Suppl.* 1974;445:25.
7. Gillquist J. Repair and reconstruction of the ACL: is it good enough? *Arthrosc J Arthrosc Relat Surg.* 1993;9(1):68–71.
8. Petersen W, Tillmann B. Structure and vascularization of the cruciate ligaments of the human knee joint. *Anat Embryol.* 1999;200(3):325–334.
9. Schreck PJ, Kitabayashi LR, Amiel D, Akeson WH, Woods VL. Integrin display increases in the wounded rabbit medial collateral ligament but not the wounded anterior cruciate ligament. *J Orthopaed Res.* 1995;13(2):174–183.
10. Witkowski J, Yang L, Wood DJ, Sung KLP. Migration and healing of ligament cells under inflammatory conditions. *J Orthopaed Res.* 1997;15(2):269–277.

11. Steiner ME, Murray MM, Rodeo SA. Strategies to improve anterior cruciate ligament healing and graft placement. *Am J Sports Med.* 2008;36(1):176–189.

12. Hirzinger C, Tauber M, Korntner S, et al. ACL injuries and stem cell therapy. *Archiv Orthopaed Trauma Surg.* 2014;134(11):1573–1578.

13. Fu FH, Bennett CH, Lattermann C, Ma CB. Current trends in anterior cruciate ligament reconstruction. Part 1: biology and biomechanics of reconstruction. *Am J Sports Med.* 1999;27(6):821–830.

14. Muller B, Bowman KF, Bedi A. ACL graft healing and biologics. *Clin Sports Med.* 2013;32(1):93–109.

15. Cameron M, Buchgraber A, Passler H, et al. The natural history of the anterior cruciate ligament-deficient knee: changes in synovial fluid cytokine and keratan sulfate concentrations. *Am J Sports Med.* 1997;25(6):751–754.

16. Romano VM, Graf BK, Keene JS, Lange RH. Anterior cruciate ligament reconstruction the effect of tibial tunnel placement on range of motion. *Am J Sports Med.* 1993;21(3):415–418.

17. Zastawna E, Drewniak W, Powierza W, Rość D, Michalski A, Kotschy M. Post-traumatic plasminogenesis in intraarticular exudate in the knee joint. *Med Sci Monit.* 2002;8(5):CR371-CR8.

18. Andersen RB, Gormsen J. Fibrin dissolution in synovial fluid. *Scand J Rheumatol.* 1987;16(1):319–333. https://doi.org/10.3109/03009747009165385. Epub 1987/01/01. PubMed PMID: 20144123.

19. Harner CD, Baek GH, Vogrin TM, Carlin GJ, Kashiwaguchi S, Woo SL. Quantitative analysis of human cruciate ligament insertions. *Arthrosc J Arthrosc Relat Surg.* 1999;15(7):741–749.

20. Indelicato PA. Non-operative treatment of complete tears of the medial collateral ligament of the knee. *JBJS.* 1983;65(3):323–329.

21. Frank C, Woo S-Y, Amiel D, Harwood F, Gomez M, Akeson W. Medial collateral ligament healing: a multidisciplinary assessment in rabbits. *Am J Sports Med.* 1983;11(6):379–389.

22. Proffen BL, Sieker JT, Murray MM. Bio-enhanced repair of the anterior cruciate ligament. *Arthrosc J Arthrosc Relat Surg.* 2015;31(5):990–997. https://doi.org/10.1016/j.arthro.2014.11.016. PubMed PMID: 25595694; PubMed Central PMCID: PMCPMC4426066.

23. Sherman MF, Lieber L, Bonamo JR, Podesta L, Reiter I. The long-term followup of primary anterior cruciate ligament repair defining a rationale for augmentation. *Am J Sports Med.* 1991;19(3):243–255.

24. Strand T, Mølster A, Hordvik M, Krukhaug Y. Long-term follow-up after primary repair of the anterior cruciate ligament: clinical and radiological evaluation 15–23 years postoperatively. *Archiv Orthopaed Trauma Surg.* 2005;125(4):217–221.

25. Taylor DC, Posner M, Curl WW, Feagin JA. Isolated tears of the anterior cruciate ligament over 30-year follow-up of patients treated with arthrotomy and primary repair. *Am J Sports Med.* 2009;37(1):65–71.

26. Feagin JRJA, Curl WW. Isolated tear of the anterior cruciate ligament: 5-year follow-up study. *Am J Sports Med.* 1976;4(3):95–100.

27. Arnoczky SP, Warren RF. The microvasculature of the meniscus and its response to injury: an experimental study in the dog. *Am J Sports Med.* 1983;11(3):131–141.

28. Bray RC, Leonard CA, Salo PT. Vascular physiology and long-term healing of partial ligament tears. *J Orthopaed Res.* 2002;20(5):984–989.

29. Spindler K, Clark S, Nanney L, Davidson J. Expression of collagen and matrix metalloproteinases in ruptured human anterior cruciate ligament: an in situ hybridization study. *J Orthopaed Res.* 1996;14(6):857–861.

30. Costa-Paz M, Ayerza MA, Tanoira I, Astoul J, Muscolo DL. Spontaneous healing in complete ACL ruptures: a clinical and MRI study. *Clin Orthopaed Relat Res.* 2012;470(4):979–985.

31. Li H, Tao H, Hua Y, Chen J, Li Y, Chen S. Quantitative magnetic resonance imaging assessment of cartilage status: a comparison between young men with and without anterior cruciate ligament reconstruction. *Arthrosc J Arthrosc Relat Surg.* 2013;29(12):2012–2019.

32. Murray MM, Spindler KP, Abreu E, et al. Collagen-platelet rich plasma hydrogel enhances primary repair of the porcine anterior cruciate ligament. *J Orthop Res.* 2007;25(1):81–91.

33. Kartus J, Movin T, Karlsson J. Donor-site morbidity and anterior knee problems after anterior cruciate ligament reconstruction using autografts. *Arthroscopy.* 2001;17(9):971–980.

34. Lohmander LS, Englund PM, Dahl LL, Roos EM. The long-term consequence of anterior cruciate ligament and meniscus injuries: osteoarthritis. *Am J Sports Med.* 2007;35(10):1756–1769. https://doi.org/10.1177/0363546507307396. PubMed PMID: 17761605.

35. Barenius B, Ponzer S, Shalabi A, Bujak R, Norlén L, Eriksson K. Increased risk of osteoarthritis after anterior cruciate ligament reconstruction: a 14-year follow-up study of a randomized controlled trial. *Am J Sports Med.* 2014;42(5):1049–1057.

36. Bonfim TR, Paccola CAJ, Barela JA. Proprioceptive and behavior impairments in individuals with anterior cruciate ligament reconstructed knees. *Archiv Phys Med Rehabil.* 2003;84(8):1217–1223.

37. Devita P, Hortobagyi T, Barrier J. Gait biomechanics are not normal after anterior cruciate ligament reconstruction and accelerated rehabilitation. *Med Sci Sports Exerc.* 1998;30:1481–1488.

38. Fremerey R, Lobenhoffer P, Zeichen J, Skutek M, Bosch U, Tscherne H. Proprioception after rehabilitation and reconstruction in knees with deficiency of the anterior cruciate ligament. *Bone Joint J.* 2000;82(6):801–806.

39. Lephart SM, Kocher MS, Fu FH, Borsa PA, Harner CD. Proprioception following anterior cruciate ligament reconstruction. *J Sport Rehabil.* 1992;1(3):188–196.

40. M-w Z, Gu L, Chen Y-p, et al. Factors affecting proprioceptive recovery after anterior cruciate ligament reconstruction. *Chin Med J.* 2008;121(22):2224–2228.

41. Rodeo SA, Arnoczky SP, Torzilli PA, Hidaka C, Warren RF. Tendon-healing in a bone tunnel. A biomechanical and histological study in the dog. *J Bone Joint Surg Am Volume.* 1993;75(12):1795–1803.

42. Whiston T, Walmsley R. Some observations on the reaction of bone and tendon after tunnelling of bone and insertion of tendon. *Bone Joint J.* 1960;42(2):377–386.

43. Grana WA, Egle DM, Mahnken R, Goodhart CW. An analysis of autograft fixation after anterior cruciate ligament reconstruction in a rabbit model. *Am J Sports Med.* 1994;22(3):344–351.

44. da Silveira Franciozi CE, Ingham SJ, Gracitelli GC, Luzo MV, Fu FH, Abdalla RJ. Updates in biological therapies for knee injuries: anterior cruciate ligament. *Curr Reviews Musculoskeletal Medicine.* 2014;7(3):228–238. https://doi.org/10.1007/s12178-014-9228-9. Epub 2014/07/30. PubMed PMID: 25070265; PubMed Central PMCID: PMCPMC4596162.

45. Waryasz GR, Marcaccio S, Gil JA, Owens BD, Fadale PD. Anterior cruciate ligament repair and biologic innovations. *JBJS Rev.* 2017;5(5):e2. https://doi.org/10.2106/jbjs.rvw.16.00050. Epub 2017/05/10. PubMed PMID: 28486257.

46. Meaney Murray M, Rice K, Wright RJ, Spector M. The effect of selected growth factors on human anterior cruciate ligament cell interactions with a three-dimensional collagen-GAG scaffold. *J Orthopaed Res.* 2003;21(2):238–244. https://doi.org/10.1016/s0736-0266(02)00142-0. Epub 2003/02/06.PubMed PMID: 12568954.

47. Kimura Y, Hokugo A, Takamoto T, Tabata Y, Kurosawa H. Regeneration of anterior cruciate ligament by biodegradable scaffold combined with local controlled release of basic fibroblast growth factor and collagen wrapping. *Tissue Eng C, Methods.* 2008;14(1):47–57. https://doi.org/10.1089/tec.2007.0286. Epub 2008/05/06. PubMed PMID: 18454645.

48. Madry H, Kohn D, Cucchiarini M. Direct FGF-2 gene transfer via recombinant adeno-associated virus vectors stimulates cell proliferation, collagen production, and the repair of experimental lesions in the human ACL. *Am J Sports Med.* 2013;41(1):194–202. https://doi.org/10.1177/0363546512465840. Epub 2012/11/23. PubMed PMID: 23172005.

49. Pascher A, Steinert AF, Palmer GD, et al. Enhanced repair of the anterior cruciate ligament by in situ gene transfer: evaluation in an in vitro model. *Mol Ther.* 2004;10(2):327–336. https://doi.org/10.1016/j.ymthe.2004.03.012. Epub 2004/08/06. PubMed PMID: 15294179.

50. Ballock RT, Woo SLY, Lyon RM, Hollis JM, Akeson WH. Use of patellar tendon autograft for anterior cruciate ligament reconstruction in the rabbit: a long-term histologic and biomechanical study. *J Orthop Res.* 1989;7(4):474–485.

51. Hogan MV, Kawakami Y, Murawski CD, Fu FH. Tissue engineering of ligaments for reconstructive surgery. *Arthrosc J Arthrosc Relat Surg.* 2015;31(5):971–979.

52. Brophy RH, Kovacevic D, Imhauser CW, et al. Effect of short-duration low-magnitude cyclic loading versus immobilization on tendon-bone healing after ACL reconstruction in a rat model. *J Bone Joint Surg Am Vol.* 2011;93(4):381.

53. Gulotta LV, Kovacevic D, Ying L, Ehteshami JR, Montgomery S, Rodeo SA. Augmentation of tendon-to-bone healing with a magnesium-based bone adhesive. *Am J Sports Med.* 2008;36(7):1290–1297.

54. Petersen W, Laprell H. Insertion of autologous tendon grafts to the bone: a histological and immunohistochemical study of hamstring and patellar tendon grafts. *Knee Surg Sports Traumatol Arthrosc.* 2000;8(1):26–31.

55. Ishibashi Y, Toh S, Okamura Y, Sasaki T, Kusumi T. Graft incorporation within the tibial bone tunnel after anterior cruciate ligament reconstruction with bone-patellar tendon-bone autograft. *Am J Sports Med.* 2001;29(4):473–479.

56. Mifune Y, Matsumoto T, Takayama K, et al. Tendon graft revitalization using adult anterior cruciate ligament (ACL)-derived CD34+ cell sheets for ACL reconstruction. *Biomaterials.* 2013;34(22):5476–5487.

57. Kawakami Y, Takayama K, Matsumoto T, et al. Anterior cruciate ligament–derived stem cells transduced with BMP2 accelerate graft-bone integration after ACL reconstruction. *Am J Sports Med.* 2017;45(3):584–597.

58. Mazzocca AD, McCarthy MBR, Chowaniec DM, et al. The positive effects of different platelet-rich plasma methods on human muscle, bone, and tendon cells. *Am J Sports Med.* 2012;40(8):1742–1749.

59. Xie X, Zhao S, Wu H, et al. Platelet-rich plasma enhances autograft revascularization and reinnervation in a dog model of anterior cruciate ligament reconstruction. *J Surg Res.* 2013;183(1):214–222.

60. Silva A, Sampaio R. Anatomic ACL reconstruction: does the platelet-rich plasma accelerate tendon healing? *Knee Surg Sports Traumatol Arthrosc.* 2009;17(6):676–682.

61. Caplan AI. Adult mesenchymal stem cells for tissue engineering versus regenerative medicine. *J Cell Physiol.* 2007;213(2):341–347.

62. Caplan AI. Mesenchymal stem cells. *J Orthopaed Res.* 1991;9(5):641–650.

63. Matsumoto T, Ingham SM, Mifune Y, et al. Isolation and characterization of human anterior cruciate ligament-derived vascular stem cells. *Stem Cells Dev.* 2011;21(6):859–872.

64. Mifune Y, Matsumoto T, Ota S, et al. Therapeutic potential of anterior cruciate ligament-derived stem cells for anterior cruciate ligament reconstruction. *Cell Transplant.* 2012;21(8):1651–1665.

65. Matsumoto T, Kubo S, Sasaki K, et al. Acceleration of tendon-bone healing of anterior cruciate ligament graft using autologous ruptured tissue. *Am J Sports Med.* 2012;40(6):1296–1302.

66. Chamberlain G, Fox J, Ashton B, Middleton J. Concise review: mesenchymal stem cells: their phenotype, differentiation capacity, immunological features, and potential for homing. *Stem Cells.* 2007;25(11):2739–2749.
67. Caplan AI. Mesenchymal stem cells the past, the present, the future. *Cartilage.* 2010;1(1):6–9.
68. Hao ZC, Wang SZ, Zhang XJ, Lu J. Stem cell therapy: a promising biological strategy for tendon–bone healing after anterior cruciate ligament reconstruction. *Cell Proliferation.* 2016.
69. Caplan AI. All MSCs are pericytes? *Cell Stem Cell.* 2008;3(3):229–230.
70. Steinert AF, Kunz M, Prager P, et al. Mesenchymal stem cell characteristics of human anterior cruciate ligament outgrowth cells. *Tissue Eng A.* 2011;17(9–10):1375–1388.
71. Morito T, Muneta T, Hara K, et al. Synovial fluid-derived mesenchymal stem cells increase after intra-articular ligament injury in humans. *Rheumatology.* 2008;47(8):1137–1143.
72. Ouyang HW, Goh JC, Lee EH. Use of bone marrow stromal cells for tendon graft-to-bone healing histological and immunohistochemical studies in a rabbit model. *Am J Sports Med.* 2004;32(2):321–327.
73. Lim J-K, Hui J, Li L, Thambyah A, Goh J, Lee E-H. Enhancement of tendon graft osteointegration using mesenchymal stem cells in a rabbit model of anterior cruciate ligament reconstruction. *Arthrosc J Arthrosc Relat Surg.* 2004;20(9):899–910.
74. Soon MY, Hassan A, Hui JH, Goh JC, Lee E. An analysis of soft tissue allograft anterior cruciate ligament reconstruction in a rabbit model a short-term study of the use of mesenchymal stem cells to enhance tendon osteointegration. *Am J Sports Med.* 2007;35(6):962–971.
75. Kanazawa T, Soejima T, Noguchi K, et al. Tendon-to-bone healing using autologous bone marrow-derived mesenchymal stem cells in ACL reconstruction without a tibial bone tunnel-A histological study. *Muscles, Ligaments Tendons J.* 2014;4(2):201.
76. Lui PPY, Wong OT, Lee YW. Application of tendon-derived stem cell sheet for the promotion of graft healing in anterior cruciate ligament reconstruction. *Am J Sports Med.* 2014;42(3):681–689.
77. Oe K, Kushida T, Okamoto N, et al. New strategies for anterior cruciate ligament partial rupture using bone marrow transplantation in rats. *Stem Cells Dev.* 2011;20(4):671–679. https://doi.org/10.1089/scd.2010.0182. Epub 2010/09/03. PubMed PMID: 20809695.
78. Pittenger MF, Mackay AM, Beck SC, et al. Multilineage potential of adult human mesenchymal stem cells. *Science.* 1999;284(5411):143–147.
79. Haynesworth SE, Baber MA, Caplan AI. Cytokine expression by human marrow-derived mesenchymal progenitor cells in vitro: effects of dexamethasone and IL-1α. *J Cell Physiol.* 1996;166(3):585–592.
80. Kanaya A, Deie M, Adachi N, Nishimori M, Yanada S, Ochi M. Intra-articular injection of mesenchymal stromal cells in partially torn anterior cruciate ligaments in a rat model. *Arthrosc J Arthrosc Relat Surg.* 2007;23(6):610–617. https://doi.org/10.1016/j.arthro.2007.01.013. Epub 2007/06/15. PubMed PMID: 17560475.
81. Agung M, Ochi M, Yanada S, et al. Mobilization of bone marrow-derived mesenchymal stem cells into the injured tissues after intraarticular injection and their contribution to tissue regeneration. Knee Surgery, Sports Traumatology. *Arthroscopy.* 2006;14(12):1307–1314.
82. Centeno CJ, Pitts J, Al-Sayegh H, Freeman MD. Anterior cruciate ligament tears treated with percutaneous injection of autologous bone marrow nucleated cells: a case series. *J Pain Res.* 2015;8:437–447. https://doi.org/10.2147/jpr.s86244. Epub 2015/08/12. PubMed PMID: 26261424; PubMed Central PMCID: PMCPMC4527573.
83. Freeman JW, Empson YM, Ekwueme EC, Paynter DM, Brolinson PG. Effect of prolotherapy on cellular proliferation and collagen deposition in MC3T3-E1 and patellar tendon fibroblast populations. *Transl Res.* 2011;158(3):132–139.
84. Yoshii Y, Zhao C, Schmelzer JD, Low PA, An K-N, Amadio PC. The effects of hypertonic dextrose injection on connective tissue and nerve conduction through the rabbit carpal tunnel. *Archiv Phys Med Rehabil.* 2009;90(2):333–339.
85. Silva A, Sampaio R, Fernandes R, Pinto E. Is there a role for adult non-cultivated bone marrow stem cells in ACL reconstruction? *Knee Surg Sports Traumatol Arthrosc.* 2014;22(1):66–71.
86. Liu H, Fan H, Toh SL, Goh JC. A comparison of rabbit mesenchymal stem cells and anterior cruciate ligament fibroblasts responses on combined silk scaffolds. *Biomaterials.* 2008;29(10):1443–1453.
87. Fan H, Liu H, Wong EJ, Toh SL, Goh JC. In vivo study of anterior cruciate ligament regeneration using mesenchymal stem cells and silk scaffold. *Biomaterials.* 2008;29(23):3324–3337.
88. Fan H, Liu H, Toh SL, Goh JC. Anterior cruciate ligament regeneration using mesenchymal stem cells and silk scaffold in large animal model. *Biomaterials.* 2009;30(28):4967–4977. https://doi.org/10.1016/j.biomaterials.2009.05.048. Epub 2009/06/23. PubMed PMID: 19539988.
89. Figueroa D, Espinosa M, Calvo R, et al. Anterior cruciate ligament regeneration using mesenchymal stem cells and collagen type I scaffold in a rabbit model. Knee Surgery, Sports Traumatology. *Arthroscopy.* 2014;22(5):1196–1202.
90. Nagineni CN, Amiel D, Green MH, Berchuck M, Akeson WH. Characterization of the intrinsic properties of the anterior cruciate and medial collateral ligament cells: an in vitro cell culture study. *J Orthopaed Res.* 1992;10(4):465–475. https://doi.org/10.1002/jor.1100100402. Epub 1992/07/01. PubMed PMID: 1613622.

91. Ferreira LS, Gerecht S, Fuller J, Shieh HF, Vunjak-Novakovic G, Langer R. Bioactive hydrogel scaffolds for controllable vascular differentiation of human embryonic stem cells. *Biomaterials*. 2007;28(17):2706–2717. https://doi.org/10.1016/j.biomaterials.2007.01.021. Epub 2007/03/10. PubMed PMID: 17346788; PubMed Central PMCID: PMCPMC1903348.

92. McDevitt CA, Wildey GM, Cutrone RM. Transforming growth factor-beta1 in a sterilized tissue derived from the pig small intestine submucosa. *J Biomed Mater Res A*. 2003;67(2):637–640. https://doi.org/10.1002/jbm.a.10144. Epub 2003/10/21. PubMed PMID: 14566807.

93. Voytik-Harbin SL, Brightman AO, Kraine MR, Waisner B, Badylak SF. Identification of extractable growth factors from small intestinal submucosa. *J Cell Biochem*. 1997;67(4):478–491. Epub 1998/01/24. PubMed PMID: 9383707.

94. Badylak S, Arnoczky S, Plouhar P, et al. Naturally occurring extracellular matrix as a scaffold for musculoskeletal repair. *Clin Orthopaed Relat Res*. 1999;(367 suppl):S333–S343. Epub 1999/11/05. PubMed PMID: 10546657.

95. Leong NL, Petrigliano FA, McAllister DR. Current tissue engineering strategies in anterior cruciate ligament reconstruction. *J Biomed Mater Res A*. 2014;102(5):1614–1624. https://doi.org/10.1002/jbm.a.34820. Epub 2013/06/06. PubMed PMID: 23737190.

96. Nau T, Teuschl A. Regeneration of the anterior cruciate ligament: current strategies in tissue engineering. *World J Orthop*. 2015;6(1):127–136. https://doi.org/10.5312/wjo.v6.i1.127. PubMed PMID: 25621217; PubMed Central PMCID: PMCPMC4303781.

97. Negahi Shirazi A, Chrzanowski W, Khademhosseini A, Dehghani F. Anterior cruciate ligament: structure, injuries and regenerative treatments. *Adv Exp Med Biol*. 2015;881:161–186. https://doi.org/10.1007/978-3-319-22345-2_10. Epub 2015/11/08. PubMed PMID: 26545750.

98. Taylor SA, Khair MM, Roberts TR, DiFelice GS. Primary repair of the anterior cruciate ligament: a systematic review. *Arthrosc J Arthrosc Relat Surg*. 2015;31(11):2233–2247. https://doi.org/10.1016/j.arthro.2015.05.007. Epub 2015/07/15. PubMed PMID: 26165465.

99. Hsu SL, Liang R, Woo SL. Functional tissue engineering of ligament healing. *Sports Med Arthrosc Rehabil Ther Technol SMARTT*. 2010;2:12. https://doi.org/10.1186/1758-2555-2-12. Epub 2010/05/25. PubMed PMID: 20492676; PubMed Central PMCID: PMCPMC2879239.

100. Nguyen DT, Dellbrugge S, Tak PP, Woo SL, Blankevoort L, van Dijk NC. Histological characteristics of ligament healing after bio-enhanced repair of the transected goat ACL. *J Exp Orthopaed*. 2015;2(1):4. https://doi.org/10.1186/s40634-015-0021-5. Epub 2016/02/26. PubMed PMID: 26914872; PubMed Central PMCID: PMCPMC4544611.

101. Fisher MB, Liang R, Jung HJ, et al. Potential of healing a transected anterior cruciate ligament with genetically modified extracellular matrix bioscaffolds in a goat model. *Knee Surg Sports Traumatol Arthrosc*. 2012;20(7):1357–1365. https://doi.org/10.1007/s00167-011-1800-x. Epub 2011/12/07. PubMed PMID: 22143425.

102. Fleming BC, Magarian EM, Harrison SL, Paller DJ, Murray MM. Collagen scaffold supplementation does not improve the functional properties of the repaired anterior cruciate ligament. *J Orthopaed Res*. 2010;28(6):703–709. https://doi.org/10.1002/jor.21071. Epub 2010/01/09. PubMed PMID: 20058276; PubMed Central PMCID: PMCPMC2858260.

103. Harrison S, Vavken P, Kevy S, Jacobson M, Zurakowski D, Murray MM. Platelet activation by collagen provides sustained release of anabolic cytokines. *Am J Sports Med*. 2011;39(4):729–734. https://doi.org/10.1177/0363546511401576. Epub 2011/03/15. PubMed PMID: 21398575; PubMed Central PMCID: PMCPMC3176726.

104. Vavken P, Fleming BC, Mastrangelo AN, Machan JT, Murray MM. Biomechanical outcomes after bioenhanced anterior cruciate ligament repair and anterior cruciate ligament reconstruction are equal in a porcine model. *Arthrosc J Arthrosc Relat Surg*. 2012;28(5):672–680. https://doi.org/10.1016/j.arthro.2011.10.008. Epub 2012/01/21. PubMed PMID: 22261137; PubMed Central PMCID: PMCPMC3340462.

105. Joshi SM, Mastrangelo AN, Magarian EM, Fleming BC, Murray MM. Collagen-platelet composite enhances biomechanical and histologic healing of the porcine anterior cruciate ligament. *Am J Sports Med*. 2009;37(12):2401–2410. https://doi.org/10.1177/0363546509339915. Epub 2009/11/27. PubMed PMID: 19940313; PubMed Central PMCID: PMCPMC2856313.

106. Murray MM, Fleming BC. Use of a bioactive scaffold to stimulate anterior cruciate ligament healing also minimizes posttraumatic osteoarthritis after surgery. *Am J Sports Med*. 2013;41(8):1762–1770. https://doi.org/10.1177/0363546513483446. Epub 2013/07/17. PubMed PMID: 23857883; PubMed Central PMCID: PMCPMC3735821.

107. Petrigliano FA, McAllister DR, Wu BM. Tissue engineering for anterior cruciate ligament reconstruction: a review of current strategies. *Arthrosc J Arthrosc Relat Surg*. 2006;22(4):441–451. https://doi.org/10.1016/j.arthro.2006.01.017. Epub 2006/04/04 .PubMed PMID: 16581458.

108. MacIntosh AC, Kearns VR, Crawford A, Hatton PV. Skeletal tissue engineering using silk biomaterials. *J Tissue Eng Regen Med*. 2008;2(2–3):71–80. https://doi.org/10.1002/term.68. Epub 2008/04/03. PubMed PMID: 18383453.

109. Rockwood DN, Preda RC, Yucel T, Wang X, Lovett ML, Kaplan DL. Materials fabrication from *Bombyx mori* silk fibroin. *Nat Protocols*. 2011;6(10):1612–1631. https://doi.org/10.1038/nprot.2011.379. Epub 2011/10/01. PubMed PMID: 21959241; PubMed Central PMCID: PMCPMC3808976.

110. Altman GH, Horan RL, Weitzel P, Richmond JC. The use of long-term bioresorbable scaffolds for anterior

cruciate ligament repair. *J Am Acad Orthop Surg.* 2008;16(4):177–187. Epub 2008/04/09. PubMed PMID: 18390480.

111. Panas-Perez E, Gatt CJ, Dunn MG. Development of a silk and collagen fiber scaffold for anterior cruciate ligament reconstruction. *J Mater Sci Mater Med.* 2013;24(1):257–265. https://doi.org/10.1007/s10856-012-4781-5. PubMed PMID: 23053810.

112. Murray MM, Flutie BM, Kalish LA, et al. The bridge-enhanced anterior cruciate ligament repair (BEAR) procedure: an early feasibility cohort study. *Orthop J Sports Med.* 2016;4(11):2325967116672176. https://doi.org/10.1177/2325967116672176. Epub 2016/12/03. PubMed PMID: 27900338; PubMed Central PMCID: PMCPMC5120682.

113. Proffen BL, Perrone GS, Fleming BC, et al. Electron beam sterilization does not have a detrimental effect on the ability of extracellular matrix scaffolds to support in vivo ligament healing. *J Orthopaed Res.* 2015;33(7):1015–1023. https://doi.org/10.1002/jor.22855. Epub 2015/02/14. PubMed PMID: 25676876; PubMed Central PMCID: PMCPMC4517185.

114. Hall MP, Band PA, Meislin RJ, Jazrawi LM, Cardone DA. Platelet-rich plasma: current concepts and application in sports medicine. *J Am Acad Orthop Surg.* 2009;17(10):602–608. Epub 2009/10/02. PubMed PMID: 19794217.

115. LaPrade RF, Geeslin AG, Murray IR, et al. Biologic treatments for sports injuries II think tank-current concepts, future research, and barriers to advancement, Part 1: biologics overview, ligament injury, tendinopathy. *Am J Sports Med.* 2016;44(12):3270–3283. https://doi.org/10.1177/0363546516634674. Epub 2016/05/10. PubMed PMID: 27159318.

116. Kajikawa Y, Morihara T, Sakamoto H, et al. Platelet-rich plasma enhances the initial mobilization of circulation-derived cells for tendon healing. *J Cell Physiol.* 2008;215(3):837–845. https://doi.org/10.1002/jcp.21368. Epub 2008/01/09. PubMed PMID: 18181148.

117. Sheth U, Simunovic N, Klein G, et al. Efficacy of autologous platelet-rich plasma use for orthopaedic indications: a meta-analysis. *J Bone Joint Surg Am.* 2012;94(4):298–307. https://doi.org/10.2106/jbjs.k.00154. Epub 2012/01/14. PubMed PMID: 22241606.

118. Starantzis KA, Mastrokalos D, Koulalis D, Papakonstantinou O, Soucacos PN, Papagelopoulos PJ. The potentially positive role of PRPs in preventing femoral tunnel widening in ACL reconstruction surgery using hamstrings: a clinical study in 51 patients. *J Sports Med.* 2014;2014:789317. https://doi.org/10.1155/2014/789317. Epub 2014/01/01. PubMed PMID: 26464895; PubMed Central PMCID: PMCPMC4590903.

119. Darabos N, Haspl M, Moser C, Darabos A, Bartolek D, Groenemeyer D. Intraarticular application of autologous conditioned serum (ACS) reduces bone tunnel widening after ACL reconstructive surgery in a randomized controlled trial. *Knee Surg Sports Traumatol Arthrosc.* 2011;19(suppl 1):S36–S46. https://doi.org/10.1007/s00167-011-1458-4. Epub 2011/03/02. PubMed PMID: 21360125.

120. Di Matteo B, Loibl M, Andriolo L, et al. Biologic agents for anterior cruciate ligament healing: a systematic review. *World J Orthop.* 2016;7(9):592–603. https://doi.org/10.5312/wjo.v7.i9.592. PubMed PMID: 27672573; PubMed Central PMCID: PMCPMC5027015.

121. Orrego M, Larrain C, Rosales J, et al. Effects of platelet concentrate and a bone plug on the healing of hamstring tendons in a bone tunnel. *Arthrosc J Arthrosc Relat Surg.* 2008;24(12):1373–1380. https://doi.org/10.1016/j.arthro.2008.07.016. Epub 2008/11/29. PubMed PMID: 19038708.

122. Figueroa D, Figueroa F, Calvo R, Vaisman A, Ahumada X, Arellano S. Platelet-rich plasma use in anterior cruciate ligament surgery: systematic review of the literature. *Arthrosc J Arthrosc Relat Surg.* 2015;31(5):981–988. https://doi.org/10.1016/j.arthro.2014.11.022. PubMed PMID: 25595696.

123. Mirzatolooei F, Alamdari MT, Khalkhali HR. The impact of platelet-rich plasma on the prevention of tunnel widening in anterior cruciate ligament reconstruction using quadrupled autologous hamstring tendon: a randomised clinical trial. *Bone Joint J.* 2013;95-B(1):65–69. https://doi.org/10.1302/0301-620x.95b1.30487. Epub 2013/01/12. PubMed PMID: 23307675.

124. Silva A, Sampaio R, Pinto E. Femoral tunnel enlargement after anatomic ACL reconstruction: a biological problem?. *Knee Surg Sports Traumatol Arthrosc.* 2010;18(9):1189–1194. https://doi.org/10.1007/s00167-010-1046-z. Epub 2010/01/30. PubMed PMID: 20111952.

125. Vadala A, Iorio R, De Carli A, et al. Platelet-rich plasma: does it help reduce tunnel widening after ACL reconstruction?. *Knee Surg Sports Traumatol Arthrosc.* 2013;21(4):824–829. https://doi.org/10.1007/s00167-012-1980-z. Epub 2012/04/11. PubMed PMID: 22488012.

126. Del Torto M, Enea D, Panfoli N, Filardo G, Pace N, Chiusaroli M. Hamstrings anterior cruciate ligament reconstruction with and without platelet rich fibrin matrix. *Knee Surg Sports Traumatol Arthrosc.* 2015;23(12):3614–3622. https://doi.org/10.1007/s00167-014-3260-6. Epub 2014/09/01. PubMed PMID: 25173508.

127. Figueroa D, Melean P, Calvo R, et al. Magnetic resonance imaging evaluation of the integration and maturation of semitendinosus-gracilis graft in anterior cruciate ligament reconstruction using autologous platelet concentrate. *Arthrosc J Arthrosc Relat Surg.* 2010;26(10):1318–1325. https://doi.org/10.1016/j.arthro.2010.02.010. Epub 2010/08/31. PubMed PMID: 20800986.

128. Valenti Azcarate A, Lamo-Espinosa J, Aquerreta Beola JD, Hernandez Gonzalez M, Mora Gasque G, Valenti Nin JR. Comparison between two different platelet-rich plasma preparations and control applied during anterior cruciate ligament reconstruction. Is there any evidence to support their use? *Injury.* 2014;45(suppl 4):S36–S41.

https://doi.org/10.1016/s0020-1383(14)70008-7. Epub 2014/11/12. PubMed PMID: 25384473.

129. Vogrin M, Rupreht M, Crnjac A, Dinevski D, Krajnc Z, Recnik G. The effect of platelet-derived growth factors on knee stability after anterior cruciate ligament reconstruction: a prospective randomized clinical study. *Wien Klinische Wochenschr*. 2010;122(suppl 2):91–95. https://doi.org/10.1007/s00508-010-1340-2. Epub 2010/06/11. PubMed PMID: 20517680.

130. Rupreht M, Vogrin M, Hussein M. MRI evaluation of tibial tunnel wall cortical bone formation after platelet-rich plasma applied during anterior cruciate ligament reconstruction. *Radiol Oncol*. 2013;47(2):119–124. https://doi.org/10.2478/raon-2013-0009. Epub 2013/06/27. PubMed PMID: 23801907; PubMed Central PMCID: PMCPMC3691087.

131. Seijas R, Ares O, Catala J, Alvarez-Diaz P, Cusco X, Cugat R. Magnetic resonance imaging evaluation of patellar tendon graft remodelling after anterior cruciate ligament reconstruction with or without platelet-rich plasma. *J Orthopaedic Surg*. 2013;21(1):10–14. https://doi.org/10.1177/230949901302100105. Epub 2013/05/01. PubMed PMID: 23629979.

132. Radice F, Yanez R, Gutierrez V, Rosales J, Pinedo M, Coda S. Comparison of magnetic resonance imaging findings in anterior cruciate ligament grafts with and without autologous platelet-derived growth factors. *Arthrosc J Arthrosc Relat Surg*. 2010;26(1):50–57. https://doi.org/10.1016/j.arthro.2009.06.030. Epub 2010/02/02. PubMed PMID: 20117627.

133. Ventura A, Terzaghi C, Borgo E, Verdoia C, Gallazzi M, Failoni S. Use of growth factors in ACL surgery: preliminary study. *J Orthop Traumatol*. 2005;6(2):76–79. https://doi.org/10.1007/s10195-005-0085-6.

134. Dallo I, Chahla J, Mitchell JJ, Pascual-Garrido C, Feagin JA, LaPrade RF. Biologic approaches for the treatment of partial tears of the anterior cruciate ligament: a current concepts review. *Orthop J Sports Med*. 2017;5(1):2325967116681724. https://doi.org/10.1177/2325967116681724. PubMed PMID: 28210653; PubMed Central PMCID: PMCPMC5298533.

135. Seijas R, Ares O, Cusco X, Alvarez P, Steinbacher G, Cugat R. Partial anterior cruciate ligament tears treated with intraligamentary plasma rich in growth factors. *World J Orthop*. 2014;5(3):373–378. https://doi.org/10.5312/wjo.v5.i3.373. Epub 2014/07/19. PubMed PMID: 25035842; PubMed Central PMCID: PMCPMC4095032.

136. Gobbi A, Karnatzikos G, Sankineani SR, Petrera M. Biological augmentation of ACL refixation in partial lesions in a group of athletes: results at the 5-year follow-up. *Tech Orthop*. 2013;28(2):180–184. https://doi.org/10.1097/BTO.0b013e318294ce44. PubMed PMID: 00013611-201306000-00011.

FURTHER READING

1. Mutsuzaki H, Sakane M, Nakajima H, et al. Calcium-phosphate-hybridized tendon directly promotes regeneration of tendon-bone insertion. *J Biomed Mater Res A*. 2004;70(2):319–327.

CHAPTER 11

Psychology of Return to Play After Anterior Cruciate Ligament Injury

JAMES D. DOORLEY, MA • MELISSA N. WOMBLE, PHD

Anterior cruciate ligament (ACL) injuries occur frequently in young and otherwise healthy athletes, making return to sport a primary concern.[1] Although some athletes may return to sport as early as 4–6 months after ACL reconstruction (ACLR),[2] they are typically expected to return to preinjury levels of sport participation approximately 1 year after operation. However, research indicates that many athletes do not return to sport as quickly as anticipated. A study of 503 competitive athletes rehabilitating from ACLR found that only 63% returned to some form of sport activity at 12 months after operation, with only 33% attempting competitive sports.[3] Notably, men were significantly more likely to return to their sport than women. In a subsequent study, 122 athletes from the same sample who did not return to their preinjury level of sport at 12 months were assessed again at 24 months after operation.[4] While the majority of athletes returned to some form of sport participation between 12 and 24 months (91%), only 66% of these athletes were participating in their sport at the time of evaluation. Of those athletes, only 41% reported playing at their preinjury level and the remaining 25% playing at a lower level. Together, these studies show that a meaningful percentage of athletes do not return to sport at 1 year, or even 2 years after operation.

It would be logical to assume that lower-than-expected return to play rates are a function of poor physical outcomes from surgery or suboptimal objective knee functioning, but the data suggest otherwise. In fact, findings generally point to a discrepancy between the effectiveness of ACLR in restoring objective knee functioning and the percentage of ACL-repaired athletes who successfully return to their preinjury levels of sport participation. Studies suggest that between 20% and 50% of athletes do not return to their same sport after surgery despite successful physical rehabilitation.[2,5] In the sample of 503 athletes noted earlier, 93% showed "nearly normal" to "normal" knee functioning on the International Knee Documentation Committee knee evaluation form at a 12-month follow-up. Objective measures showed that 84% of athletes had a hop-test

limb symmetry index of 85% or greater. A meta-analysis of 48 studies and a total of 5770 participants found that by a postoperative mean of 36.7 months, only 44% of athletes returned to competitive sports, although 85%–90% achieved normal or nearly normal objective knee functioning.[6]

When looking solely at the abovementioned findings, the mechanism driving this discrepancy seems unclear. What *is* clear is that physical readiness is an unreliable indicator of successful return to sport, despite an abundance of research attention given to physical aspects of ACLR recovery.[7,8] An implicit assumption in this literature is that physical and psychological readiness to return to sport follow the same trajectory, but a growing body of research suggests this is often not the case.[3] Although many athletes believe that ACLR is an essential path toward return to sport, athletes are often psychologically ill-prepared for surgery and the rehabilitation process.[9] One study assessed 87 athletes 12 months after ACLR and found no significant differences in objective knee functioning between the athletes who returned to sport by 12 months and those who did not.[10] However, athletes who had not returned to sport reported significantly lower psychological readiness to return to sport at 6 and 12 months after ACLR. Another study assessed 187 athletes 12 months after undergoing ACLR to determine the role of psychological factors in return to sport.[11] At 12 months, only 31% of athletes returned to preinjury levels of sport participation. Those who did not return showed significantly lower psychological readiness to return to sport, were more fearful of reinjuring their knee, had stronger beliefs that rehabilitation was out of their control (i.e., external locus of control), and estimated that it would take significantly longer for them to return to sport when asked preoperatively and 4 months postoperatively. Other studies have yielded similar results at 12 months and 3–4 years after ACLR,[12,13] showing that athletes who did not return to sport were more fearful of reinjuring their knee, experienced more negative emotions, and had lower self-confidence.

ACL Injuries in Female Athletes. https://doi.org/10.1016/B978-0-323-54839-7.00011-7

The biopsychosocial model of sport injury rehabilitation suggests that a number of psychological factors in the domains of personality, cognition, and behavior influence sport injury rehabilitation and return to play outcomes.[14] Literature reviews have outlined the most prominent psychological factors in each of these domains.[15-17] These include mood-related factors such as depression, performance anxiety, and fear of reinjury; cognitive factors such as self-confidence, motivation/self-determination, athletic identity, and perceptions of control over one's recovery (i.e., locus of control); and behavioral factors such as compliance and social support. While these mechanisms and their relevance to return to sport outcomes have been noted in prior research, their relevance for female athletes specifically has received insufficient attention, despite the consensus that female athletes have worse return to sport outcomes than men following ACLR.[3,18] For example, a meta-analysis with pooled data across 18 studies showed that men had greater odds of returning to preinjury levels of sport participation, as well as any level of competitive sport participation, than women following ACLR.[6] Researchers have speculated that neuromuscular deficiencies among female athletes underlie these gender differences.[19] However, this conflicts with the findings mentioned earlier, demonstrating the predictive potency of psychological factors above and beyond physical factors in post-ACL return to sport outcomes. Thus, if psychological factors play a primary role, it would logically follow that these factors are more prominent among female athletes. In the following, we review each of the primary psychological factors relevant for return to sport. Where research exists, we point out the unique ways these psychological factors manifest among women and impede return to sport. Next, we briefly review empirically supported measures that can be easily integrated into clinical practice to assess these psychological factors. Finally, we outline the ways in which sport psychologists and other mental health professionals can help patients overcome the psychological barriers to ACL rehabilitation and improve return to sport outcomes.

MOOD DISTURBANCE

The psychological impact of ACL injuries and other sports injuries has been well-documented throughout the sport psychology literature. Much of the early research in this area focused on general mood-related factors including "mood disturbance" or "psychological distress." Other studies have focused on changes in "affect" or "emotions" after ACL injury. Unfortunately, the terms used in prior orthopedic and sport psychology studies are often used interchangeably and inconsistently with intended meanings from their origins in psychological research. We will use the term "mood disturbance," as it captures the various forms of mood changes investigated by prior studies, including decreases in positive mood states and increases in negative mood states. Beyond the mere presence of mood disturbance following ACL injuries, studies have examined the temporal dynamics of mood disturbance across the rehabilitation trajectory. This research suggests that mood disturbance follows a "U"-shaped curve over time, with the greatest mood disturbances occurring shortly after ACLR and again at 6-month follow-up.[20]

Mood disturbance is likely to be prominent at both time points for different reasons. Following ACLR, athletes may be struggling to adjust after the injury itself, experiencing pain from surgery, suffering from lack of sleep, and worrying about the course of their recovery. One study by Brewer and colleagues[21] assessed daily mood disturbance in the early stages of ACLR rehabilitation for 42 consecutive days. Results showed that on average, negative mood was associated with daily pain and daily stress and was more common among individuals higher on neuroticism (i.e., the tendency to react to stressful or uncertain circumstances with higher levels of negative affect).[22] Negative mood significantly decreased over the course of the study, which appears to be inconsistent with the "U"-shaped curve suggested in prior research. However, patients were only followed for 42 days and were not observed at the 6-month mark, when mood disturbance is expected to increase.[20] Interestingly, the greatest decreases in negative mood occurred in individuals with stronger athletic identities (i.e., those who strongly identified with the role of being an athlete) and those who were less optimistic.[23] A closer review of findings showed that higher athletic identity was associated with greater negative mood on average in the early stages of recovery, but with more of a decline in negative mood later on. It may be that individuals with stronger athletic identities are affected more negatively immediately after ACL injury because a core feature of their identity has been threatened. However, they may display more emotional resilience (in terms of decreased negative affect) as rehabilitation progresses and they perceive greater progress toward regaining their sense of identity through sport participation. Regarding the optimism findings, those who were more optimistic had lower negative mood in the early stages of recovery, whereas those who were less optimistic initially had higher negative mood but may have been more emotionally reactive to their objective progress, resulting in greater decreases in negative mood as they began to see more positive results later in their recovery.

Mood disturbance at the 6-month milestone may be a product of protracted recovery, an inability to return to sport as desired, fear of reinjuring one's knee, and/or performing poorly upon being cleared for competitive sport.[20] While mood disturbance in the early stages of rehabilitation may present as sadness and generally low mood, the nature of mood disturbance may alter as recovery and return to sport are imminent. It is suspected that mood disturbance at 6 months is being driven by an imminent return to sport (e.g., anxiety) or a failure to return to sport as expected (e.g., sadness); however, this is difficult to fully determine, as most previous studies have not examined return to sport outcomes at the 6-month mark.[20] Morrey and colleagues[20] suggest that competitive athletes experience significantly greater mood disturbance upon receiving medical clearance to return to sport than recreational athletes. One explanation for these findings is that competitive athletes exhibit greater anxiety about whether they will return to preinjury levels of sport performance, as they were performing at higher levels before injury than recreational athletes and likely have greater pressures to return to this level (e.g., monetary and career-related incentives).

Considerations for Women

Negative or depressed mood is one of the most common reactions to sports injuries.[14] Thus the prevalence of/risk for depression among women relative to men is worth discussing. A large body of evidence suggests that the prevalence of depression is significantly greater among females throughout adolescence and adulthood,[24] with females being approximately twice as likely to experience depression throughout this period than males.[25] Although major depression may be equally heritable in men and women,[26] women may experience certain life stressors more frequently than men and display psychological and biological reactions to stress that increase the risk for depression.[25] Although a large body of research has examined gender differences in depressive symptoms, far less attention has been given to these issues among athletes, and even less among athletes after experiencing sports injuries such as an ACL rupture.

One prospective study examined mood changes before and after injury among 276 athletes and found that both depression and anger increased significantly after injury, but these changes were roughly equivalent for men and women.[27] As a caveat, only 36 of the 276 athletes sustained a sports injury during the course of the study, resulting in insufficient power to detect the potential moderating effects of gender that may have actually been present. Another study used a self-report symptom checklist and a diagnostic clinical interview to assess depression at 1 week, 1 month, and 3 months following injury among male and female athletes with and without sports injuries.[28] Results showed that on average, women had significantly greater depressive symptoms per the clinical interview than males, regardless of injury status. However, depression scores on the clinical interview for men and women with injuries were virtually equal. These data coincide with other studies suggesting that, on average, female athletes experience greater depressive symptoms than males.[29,30] Taken together, it is unclear whether women experience greater levels of mood disturbance, and depressed mood specifically, following ACL injuries but female athletes (and females in general) appear to be more prone to depression than male athletes. Medical professionals should be aware of this risk when working with female athletes with ACL injuries.

Measures

Measures such as the Emotional Response of Athletes to Injury Questionnaire (ERAIQ)[31] and the Profile of Mood States (POMS)[32] have been widely used in the sport psychology literature to assess mood disturbance due to injury recovery. The ERAIQ assesses injured athletes' psychosocial responses to injury and is intended to be administered by a medical professional in an interview format, although the ERAIQ has been adapted as a self-report questionnaire in prior research.[33] The ERAIQ was initially developed through clinical interviews with injured athletes and yields a range of both qualitative and quantitative information about the injured athlete's emotional response to injury as well as other relevant information for determining risk for mood disturbance. For example, the ERAIQ asks athletes to what extent they identify themselves as an athlete, what their goals are in their sport, how the injury happened, whether they are encouraged in their sport by significant others, what emotions they are feeling, and how motivated they are to return to sport.[31]

The POMS has been widely used as a measure of psychological distress among healthy individuals, patients with medical or psychiatric diagnoses, and athletes.[34,35] The original POMS is composed of 65 adjectives (e.g., "angry," "tense," "lively," "hopeless"). Patients rate the extent to which these adjectives describe them during the past week using a 1–5 Likert scale. The POMS also yields scores on six subscales:

fatigue-inertia, vigor-activity, tension-anxiety, depression-dejection, anger-hostility, and confusion-bewilderment. Multiple condensed versions of the POMS have been published and psychometrically validated with large samples of medical patients, including the Brief POMS,[36] which contains 11 of the original items and yields an overall distress score, and the POMS Short Form (POMS-SF),[37] which contains 37 of the original POMS items and yields an overall distress score and retains the six subscale scores from the original POMS. Data suggest that the psychometric properties of the POMS-SF subscales are very similar to those of the original POMS and, therefore, may be an ideal alternative for medical professionals looking to obtain the same information as the original POMS, but with a shorter scale.[31] Various versions of the POMS have been used to evaluate mood disturbance among athletes rehabilitating from ACLR.[20,38] The POMS can be an effective tool for measuring athletes' mood disturbance during ACLR rehabilitation, but mood disturbance is not necessarily predictive of poor return to sport outcomes. For example, one study found that mood disturbance as measured by the POMS was significantly associated with sport confidence but not with return to sport rates.[39] However, fear of reinjury was significantly associated with return to sport. These data suggest that while mood disturbance may negatively impact an athlete's subjective experience during recovery, other factors such as fear and anxiety may play a more prominent role in objective return to sport outcomes.

ANXIETY AND FEAR OF REINJURY

Fear of reinjuring one's knee and anxiety about the consequences of doing so are the most frequently reported psychological difficulties among athletes returning to sport after ACL injuries. The term "fear of reinjury" is often used interchangeably with "kinesiophobia" in the sport psychology literature, and although both constructs are closely linked, there are semantic differences between the two. Kinesiophobia has been defined as an irrational and debilitating fear of physical movement resulting from a feeling of vulnerability to painful injury or reinjury.[40,41] In this way, the irrational fear of movement known as kinesiophobia stems from a maladaptive thought process in which the injured person associates movement with a strong likelihood of reinjuring oneself (i.e., fear of reinjury). As these constructs are often used synonymously, we will use the term fear of reinjury for ease of interpretation.

Early studies have linked fear of reinjury to impaired physical performance following injury and avoidance of physical or sporting activities.[41,42] This avoidance can behaviorally manifest in the form of hesitation/holding back, giving less than maximal effort, being wary of situations that may cause injury, and ultimately underutilizing the injured body part in sports to the detriment of performance quality and self-confidence.[43] Several studies have examined the role of fear of reinjury in rehabilitation and return to sport outcomes for athletes. Kvist and colleagues[12] assessed fear of reinjury in a sample of 62 athletes who had undergone ACLR approximately 3–4 years prior. Results showed that 47% of athletes had not returned to preinjury levels of sport participation (there were no gender differences in return to sport rates) and nearly a quarter (24%) of these athletes cited fear of reinjury as the primary reason for not returning to sport. In contrast, patients who did return to preinjury levels of sport participation had lower levels of fear of reinjury on average.

In another study, 135 athletes (ranging from recreational to professional) were interviewed 12–25 months following ACLR to assess return to sport rates and reasons for not returning.[40] Results indicated that 54% of athletes did not return to their preinjury level of sport participation. Among the nonreturners, 52% cited fear of reinjury as the primary reason, which was the second most common reason cited after persistent knee pain (63%). Furthermore, of the 50 athletes who reported that they did not return to sport because of persistent knee pain, 25 (50%) athletes also cited fear of reinjury, suggesting a possible link between persistent pain at the injury site and a fear of reinjury. There were no significant differences in reporting fear of reinjury by gender. In a larger study of 209 athletes who had already returned to sport following ACLR, results showed that athletes who returned to their preinjury levels of sport participation had significantly less fear of reinjury than those who did not.[44] This suggests that fear of reinjury may predict more granular differences in levels of sport participation among returning athletes, in addition to whether athletes return to sport in general. Other research suggests that fear of reinjury may be a particularly potent predictor of return to sport compared with other relevant predictors. One study assessed 49 athletes 1 year after ACLR and found that fear of reinjury, pain catastrophizing, and negative affect were all negatively associated with athletes' confidence in their ability to return to sport. However, only fear of reinjury significantly predicted whether athletes had actually returned to sport 1 year after surgery.[39]

Taken together, these studies suggest that fear of reinjury is one of the primary reasons why athletes fail to return to sport following ACLR.

Considerations for Women

The fear and avoidance model of musculoskeletal pain states that when individuals perceive pain as a threat following musculoskeletal injury, they begin to catastrophize about their pain (i.e., assume that their pain indicates a potential catastrophic problem, or will lead to catastrophic consequences) and become fearful of movement as a function of a broader fear of reinjury. These psychological changes can then lead to decreased use, deconditioning, depression, disability, and increased pain levels.[45] This suggests that at the core of fear of reinjury is a tendency to perceive disproportionate levels of threat in one's environment and overestimate the likelihood of catastrophic events. In other words, neuroticism and a propensity toward anxiety is theoretically associated with fear of reinjury.

An abundance of research indicate that women report higher levels of fear and anxiety and are at greater risk for developing anxiety disorders than men.[46] These gender differences are apparent in children as young as 9 years old,[47,48] adolescents,[45] and adults.[46] It may be that gender differences in maladaptive cognitive appraisals underlie differential levels of anxiety among men and women.[49,50] For example, women are more likely to overestimate the likelihood of harm and danger in their environments,[51,52] which can foster anxiety. From an evolutionary perspective, this may have once been an adaptive trait for women, increasing hypervigilance toward possible dangers that may threaten their offspring.[53] Other research suggests that women tend to perceive that they have less control over their environments and have higher levels of rumination (i.e., thoughts or behaviors that cause a maladaptive focus on feelings of depression or negative affect), which can exacerbate anxiety.[25,54-56] Given these findings, it would make sense that women are at greater risk for developing maladaptive cognitive appraisals of their injured knee that could lead to anxiety and fear of reinjury, and subsequently, difficulties returning to sport successfully. As noted earlier, pooled data across 18 studies suggest that women are less likely to return to preinjury levels of sport participation following ACL injury compared with men.[6] Gender differences in risk for anxiety problems may mediate this association. Future research should aim to evaluate fear of reinjury as a potential mechanism driving return to sport discrepancies among men and women.

Measures

The ERAIQ (see the section "Mood Disturbance") assesses a range of emotional responses to athletic injuries, including fear of reinjury.[31,33] The ERAIQ evaluates fear of reinjury with a single item (i.e., "Do you have fears about returning to sport?") to which athletes respond "Yes" or "No," with the option of providing a free qualitative response if the answer is "Yes". Although the ERAIQ may provide useful clinical information, other quantitative self-report measures show stronger psychometric properties in evaluating fear of reinjury using several items. These include the Return to Sport After Serious Injury Questionnaire (RSSIQ)[57] and the Tampa Scale for Kinesiophobia (TSK).[41]

The RSSIQ is a 21-item self-report measure designed for use after athletes have already returned to sport following injury. The scale measures athletes' psychological experience of returning to sport, including levels of concern/anxiety about their injury and their performance (e.g., "my belief in myself has been lower," "my fear of reinjury has interfered with performances," "my anxiety about competing has been greater") and the extent to which they have gained a renewed, positive perspective on their sport (e.g., "my appreciation of sport has been greater," "my motivation for sport success has been greater," "my mental toughness has been better").

The TSK is a 17-item self-report questionnaire that has been used to assess fear of movement (e.g., "It's really not safe for a person with a condition like mine to be physically active") and fear of reinjury (e.g., "pain always means I have injured my body") in a variety of patient populations such as those with lower-back pain,[54] chronic neck pain,[55] and sports injuries including ACL ruptures.[2,58,59] High scores on the TSK (indicative of high levels of fear of movement and reinjury) have been found to predict poor return to sport outcomes among athletes recovering from ACLR.[11,12,40] The original TSK shows acceptable psychometric properties, whereas a shortened version of the TSK, the TSK-11, excludes six of the psychometrically weakest items from the original TSK and demonstrates similar validity and reliability while being faster to complete.[42,60]

LOCUS OF CONTROL, SELF-EFFICACY, AND SELF-CONFIDENCE

Research on self-efficacy and self-confidence in sports injury rehabilitation evolved from earlier work on health locus of control in the 1970s and 80s. Health locus of control is defined as the extent to which individuals attribute their health to their actions or to the influence of external agents.[61] Individuals with an *internal* health locus of control believe that positive health results emerge from their willpower and sustained efforts, whereas individuals with an *external* health locus of control believe that fate, luck, powerful others, or even supernatural occurrences influence their health outcomes.[61] Much of the research on health locus of control was focused on how patients behave, adapt, and adhere to treatments following medical diagnoses. This research suggested that individuals with an internal locus of control who tend to believe that their efforts will produce results experience greater reductions in physical pain and psychological discomfort during treatment.[61] These individuals tend to have greater knowledge about their illness and greater success with smoking cessation and weight loss interventions.[62–64]

Data also suggest that two types of external loci of control exist: the belief that health outcomes are up to chance and the belief that health outcomes are dictated by more powerful others (e.g., doctors).[61] Those who believe their health outcomes are up to chance believe that their behaviors have no effect on their health, but rather other factors such as fate or their environment dictate their health (e.g., genetics, weather, germs, etc.). Those who believe their health is determined by more powerful people tend to make more frequent visits to the doctor and be more reliant on their doctor's advice. While these individuals may be less likely to take independent action and actively seek out information about their illness/injury,[65] they may also adhere more strictly to doctors' prescribed treatment regimens (or a physical therapist's prescribed at-home exercises) owing to the belief that one's doctor is the only authority on one's health. Other research has supported the notion that a more general external health locus of control can be beneficial in certain contexts, such as those in which patients truly lack control over their health (e.g., patients diagnosed with cancer undergoing chemotherapy or rehabilitation[66,67]). Research has investigated the simplistic view that internal is good and external is bad but has failed to find associations between an internal locus of control and the practice of health behaviors among smokers and exercise among elderly women.[68,69] Although locus of control may play a role in ACLR rehabilitation, it is perhaps more beneficial to examine modern constructs that stemmed from the early locus of control studies, such as self-efficacy.

During the 1990s, the application of self-efficacy research to health domains became popular, as data showed that health-related self-efficacy was a stronger predictor of health behaviors than locus of control.[70] While both constructs pertain to perceptions of control, locus of control particularly relates to control over outcomes (e.g., achieving preinjury levels of performance), which are inherently less controllable than the behaviors required to achieve such outcomes, such as performing prescribed physical therapy exercises. Self-efficacy, on the other hand, relates to one's appraisal of his/her ability to successfully carry out such behaviors.[71] Early studies suggest that self-efficacy is strongly associated with the intensity and duration of effort that individuals expend when faced with problems and adverse situations. As such, self-efficacy has been explored widely in medicine as a predictor of positive recovery outcomes in the midst of challenging circumstances. Greater self-efficacy has been found to predict physical exercise among patients undergoing cardiac rehabilitation, improved functioning in patients with low-back pain, and quality of life after having a stroke.[72–74] Given the physical and psychological rigors of ACL rehabilitation, several studies have investigated associations between self-efficacy, successful rehabilitation, and return to sport following ACLR.

Research suggests that self-efficacy may be an important factor in promoting adherence to physical therapy home exercise protocols following ACLR. One study of 270 injured athletes found that greater self-efficacy was associated with greater frequency, duration, and overall quality of exercise during rehabilitation.[75] Increases in self-efficacy may also predict decreases in knee pain intensity over the first 12 weeks following ACLR.[76] Some research has examined the role of self-efficacy in predicting physical activity levels following ACLR. One study followed 38 patients with ACL injury from before surgery to 1 year after surgery and found that greater presurgery self-efficacy related to current knee functioning significantly predicted a return to preinjury levels of physical activity 1 year after surgery. Before surgery, the authors also assessed patients' self-efficacy related to their future knee functioning, which was significantly associated with positive objective knee outcomes at 1 year after surgery based on single-leg hop performance. Presurgery self-efficacy also significantly predicted improvements in subjective knee functioning 1 year after surgery.[77]

These findings suggest that greater self-efficacy predicts decreases in knee pain, successful return to preinjury levels of physical activity, and increases in subjective and objective knee functioning 1 year after ACLR, with one potential mechanism for these changes being improved adherence to prescribed home exercises throughout recovery. Of note, much of the research in this area has not focused on athlete populations specifically, but rather on general adult populations who have sustained ACL injuries.[77,78] Future research should focus on athlete populations to better understand which types of athletes exhibit the highest levels of self-efficacy before and during ACL rehabilitation and why. Some data suggest that patients' self-efficacy is determined by how they conceptualize their knee symptoms and functioning and the extent to which they believe that successful ACL rehabilitation is a direct product of their actions (i.e., internal locus of control) as opposed to being out of their control. However, determinants of self-efficacy should be explored further in athlete populations specifically because other sport-related factors may play an important role in shaping self-efficacy, including athletic performance, successful return to sport after a previous injury, and support from teammates and coaches.

Self-confidence is related to self-efficacy and has received a great deal of attention in the sport psychology literature, as it relates to sport performance and performance anxiety.[79–82] On average, injured athletes tend to have lower self-confidence than noninjured athletes, and athletes in general have less confidence in their abilities when returning to sport after injury.[43,83] While some quantitative studies have focused specifically on lack of confidence as a predictor of poor return to sport outcomes,[10] much of this evidence has come from anecdotal reports and qualitative interviews. Professional athletes have often discussed their struggles to regain self-confidence after a long hiatus from sport due to injury. Earvin "Magic" Johnson was once quoted saying, "I had lost a lot of confidence during the long layoff. And for a long time after I returned, I still held back. All I could think about was protecting my knee from another injury."[84] This quote illustrates the notion that confidence may be influenced by other psychological constructs that affect return to sport outcomes, such as fear of reinjury. Data from a qualitative 8-month longitudinal study suggest that a number of factors can negatively impact athletes' confidence after returning to sport, including injury "flare-ups," returning to sport before being fully healed, competing against more accomplished players, and the perception of not yet playing at preinjury levels.[85]

A case study by Carson and Polman[86] offers an illustrative example of the interplay between self-confidence and self-efficacy as athletes prepare to return to sport. The authors conducted semistructured interviews with one professional athlete (rugby player) every 2–3 weeks from pre-ACLR through return to sport. Content analysis of interviews during return to sport revealed that the athlete found confidence building to be his primary concern during this phase. He reported, "I took great confidence from the pre-season training and the strength in my knee. I had concerns relating to my overall fitness but the medical staff reassured me that the preparation and testing my knee had gone through meant it was healthy."[86] This statement suggests that medical professionals can play a key role in bolstering athletes' confidence in their injured knee by encouraging them to trust that the recovery process will allow them to successfully return to sport and perform well. Prior to returning to sport, the athlete engaged in intense physical training and preparation to help him realize that his knee was strong enough for competition. This further enhanced the athlete's confidence and self-efficacy by providing him with behavioral evidence that his hard work translated into results and prepared him well for competition. Of note, interviews with the athlete did not reveal any themes related to elevated fear of reinjury. Had the athlete been more fearful of reinjuring his knee, it is unlikely that he would have engaged in such rigorous physical preparation prior to competition and thus may have been less confident that his knee could withstand the rigors of competitive sport.

Considerations for Women

Gender differences in self-confidence and self-efficacy have long been a topic of discussion in psychology, dating back to the publication of *The Psychology of Sex Differences*,[87] which suggested that women exhibit lower self-confidence in achievement situations than men. This line of research became popular with regard to physical activity, culminating in a meta-analysis by Lirgg[88] that suggested that across a number of studies, men tend to have higher self-efficacy in physical tasks than women, with a moderate effect size of .40. However, it would of course be inaccurate to conclude that *all* women have lower self-efficacy than men, or that differences manifest across all physical/sport-related contexts. Some research suggests that the nature of the physical task moderates these gender differences. For example, men have been found to report higher self-confidence in sports that are more traditionally masculine, such as football and hockey, whereas women report higher self-confidence in traditionally feminine sports, such as ballet.[89,90] When it comes to more traditionally gender-neutral sports, such as swimming, men and women have reported comparable levels of self-confidence.[89] However, gender norms in sports have evolved over the years, making a more modern replication of these results important.

If gender differences in self-confidence with physical tasks do hinge at least partially on perceptions of the masculinity/femininity of the task at hand, it is perhaps unlikely that we would see gender differences in self-efficacy during ACL rehabilitation, what many would presume to be a gender-neutral task. However, a number of factors could account for potential gender differences. For example, data suggest that men tend to overestimate their abilities compared with women and women may be socialized to be more modest than men.[88,91] Data also suggest that men tend to underestimate task difficulty or complexity compared with women, even on tasks they have never attempted before.[79] Thus when compared with women, it may be that men overestimate their abilities to successfully complete prescribed exercises during rehabilitation and underestimate the difficulties involved with making a successful return to sport. One study examined gender differences in knee-related self-efficacy over a 1-year span after ACL injury and found that women had significantly lower preoperative self-efficacy than men.[78] As other works suggest that preoperative self-efficacy predicts subjective and objective knee functioning at 1-year follow-up, low self-efficacy may be one mechanism driving return to sport difficulties among women. However, the extent to which self-efficacy is associated with actual return to sport rates is unclear. Future research should explore the role of self-efficacy in return to sport outcomes among female athletes with ACL injuries relative to males, with hopes of understanding whether, how, and when female athletes' self-efficacy impedes a positive return to sport outcomes.

Measures

There are several validated self-report measures that assess self-confidence/self-efficacy during recovery from sports injuries. These include the Self-Efficacy for Rehabilitation Outcomes Scale (SER)[92] and the Knee Self-Efficacy Scale (K-SES).[93] To our knowledge, there is one validated scale with items that assess athletes' confidence in their ability to successfully return to sports, namely, the ACL Return to Sport After Injury Scale (ACL-RSI).[13]

The SER is a useful scale for athletes rehabilitating from ACLR and includes 12 items that assess patients' beliefs about their ability to perform behaviors typical in physical rehabilitation from knee or hip surgery.[94] Items on the SER ask patients about their beliefs in being able to successfully perform more difficult tasks, with earlier items assessing patients' beliefs in their ability to stretch their leg and later items assessing patients' beliefs in their ability to walk successfully.

One advantage of the SER is that it explicitly taps into rehabilitation self-efficacy when patients are experiencing pain or psychological distress (e.g., "I believe I can do my therapy regardless of the amount of pain I am experiencing").

The K-SES has been used to assess patients perceived self-efficacy related to knee functioning and has been used specifically among patients recovering from ACL injuries.[93] The K-SES consists of 22 items that evaluate four domains of knee self-efficacy: daily activities, sports activities, knee function tasks, and knee function tasks in the future. Psychometric data suggest that the K-SES measures two distinct factors: self-efficacy related to current knee performance/functioning and self-efficacy related to future knee performance/functioning.[93] Both factors of the K-SES may be of interest to medical professionals who want to obtain information on both their patients' current knee self-efficacy at specific time points throughout rehabilitation (preoperative, postoperative, 3 months, 6 months, etc.) and their patients' predictions about what their future knee functioning will be at the time of medical clearance and return to sport. Using the K-SES at multiple time points could also allow for analysis of how well patients' predictions about their future knee self-efficacy upon medical clearance (e.g., assessed pre- or postoperatively) match their actual knee self-efficacy once the patient is medically cleared.

The ACL-RSI was designed to assess the psychological impact of returning to sport following ACLR.[13] The ACL-RSI evaluates three facets of psychological responses when returning to sports: emotions (e.g., "Are you nervous about playing your sport," "Are you fearful of reinjuring your knee by playing your sport?"), confidence in sport performance (e.g., "Are you confident that you can perform at your previous level of sport participation?"), and appraisals of risk associated with returning to sport (e.g., "Do you think you are likely to reinjure your knee by participating in your sport?"). Items in the emotion facets are primarily related to fear of reinjury and nervousness/anxiety, as these are among the most commonly reported emotional responses. Items from both the emotion and confidence facets were adapted from another validated scale that assesses quality of life among individuals with chronic ACL deficiencies.[95] Notably, scores on the ACL-RSI 6 and 12 months after surgery have been shown to significantly predict which athletes successfully return to sport at 12 months, above and beyond scores on the ERAIQ (see the measures of mood disturbance mentioned earlier).[10]

MOTIVATION AND SELF-DETERMINATION

In order for athletes to successfully return to sport, they must possess the necessary motivation to persist through a psychologically taxing rehabilitation protocol for 6–12 months or more. A number of studies have cited motivation as a key determinant for adhering to prescribed treatment protocols.[96,97] Motivation is positively associated with attendance at physical therapy sessions, completion of prescribed treatments/home exercise protocols, and self-rated adherence among patients with sports injuries and ACL injuries specifically.[14,98,99] However, according to the self-determination theory (SDT),[100] only certain forms of motivation may lead to positive rehabilitation and return to sport outcomes. SDT posits that behavior can be motivated/regulated by both external and internal sources (i.e., extrinsic and intrinsic motivation). These sources can be ordered along a continuum in terms of how autonomous or self-determined one's behaviors are. Behaviors characterized by extrinsic motivation can take four different forms, ordered from least autonomous to most autonomous: external regulation, introjected regulation, identified regulation, and integrated regulation.

In this model, the lowest level of self-determination is characterized by behaviors that are undertaken due to pressure from external forces, such as significant others.[101] In sports, athletes may experience pressure to return from family or friends, romantic partners, coaches, teammates, athletic trainers, staff members, fans, and the media (especially for professional athletes). Some athletes may internalize these pressures, even when they are no longer present (introjected regulation). For example, athletes may be motivated to return to sports out of guilt because they are worried about disappointing significant others and may feel relieved after returning to sports, believing they have gained approval from these significant others. Next, behaviors may be undertaken because of their importance or usefulness (identified regulation). Some athletes recovering from ACLR may view their prescribed at-home exercises to be particularly important for recovery or may believe that it is important to return to sport so they can actively contribute to their team. The most autonomous form of extrinsic motivation is integrated regulation, whereby individuals engage in a behavior not only because it is perceived important but also because it is in line with their core values. For example, athletes may be motivated to return to sport because they identify with the role of being a competitive athlete on a fundamental level and being held out of competition obscures their sense of purpose in life. Finally, in order for behaviors to be internally regulated, individuals must engage in a behavior simply for the pleasure and enjoyment that the given behavior brings them, without any sort of

reinforcement. This is known as intrinsic motivation. Integrated regulation is characterized by engaging in behaviors that bring about outcomes consistent with core values, whereas intrinsic motivation is characterized by engaging in behaviors simply for the sake of the interest and enjoyment of the activity itself. For example, some athletes may have a deep passion for their sport and feel engaged and alive when they are competing. When these athletes are injured, they are not motivated to adhere to prescribed treatments and return to sport because of external pressures or rewards, but rather they simply want to experience the enjoyment that playing their sport once brought them.

Indeed, studies suggest that more autonomous forms of motivation during rehabilitation are associated with greater adherence to prescribed treatments among patients with a range of medical conditions.[102] However, for individuals to be autonomously motivated, SDT suggests that three basic psychological needs must be satisfied, which are fundamental for effective functioning and psychological health: the need for autonomy (the perception that one's behaviors are one's own choice), competence (a sense of proficiency or effectiveness in the activities one engages in), and relatedness (a sense of connectedness or belonging in one's social world).[100] If these needs are met, athletes may be more autonomously motivated to return to sport and thus be more likely to engage in prescribed treatments and home exercises. If the satisfaction of basic psychological needs is thwarted, athletes may experience apathy, alienation, lack of direction, or a lack of responsibility,[103] which can negatively impact their adherence and motivation during rehabilitation. When returning to sport after a serious injury, many athletes are deprived of their autonomy, competence, and relatedness for various reasons. As noted earlier, athletes returning to sport may struggle to do so autonomously because of external pressures or incentives. Some research suggests that these external incentives can undermine autonomous motivation and make tasks that were once intrinsically motivated less rewarding.[100] Returning athletes may struggle to regain their technical abilities and their physical competency, as they worry about how and whether their body will stand up to the physical demands of their sport following an injury.[104] These worries may be exacerbated for athletes who have avoided physical activity for fear of reinjury. For many athletes, injury also means alienation from their teammates, coaches, fellow competitors, and other key social support figures, implying that injuries can thwart feelings of relatedness in athletes.[85]

Qualitative research has explored the role of basic psychological needs in athletes' motivation to return to sport. Podlog and Eklund[85] interviewed 12 elite athletes returning to sport after injury to determine the extent to which psychological needs satisfaction played a role in the athletes' perspectives on their recovery over time. Their sample consisted of two track athletes, one netball player, one field hockey player, and one ice hockey player. Results revealed that themes related to SDT were prominent for athletes throughout the return to sport process. Regarding autonomy, athletes reported that having the freedom to return to sport at their own pace was beneficial in alleviating stress. This is consistent with past research by the same authors, suggesting that an enhanced sense of autonomy is beneficial for athletes returning from injury.[57,105] Multiple themes emerged with regard to competence, as athletes reported a number of competency goals for returning back to sport, including improving skills, regaining pre-injury performance capabilities, and achieving personal bests. This suggests that giving athletes ample opportunities to work toward and achieve personal goals may help satisfy needs for competence. Regarding relatedness, some athletes reported feeling isolated during rehabilitation and separated from their teammates and training partners. However, athletes noted that they felt driven to return to sport in order to reconnect with teammates/coaches, to feel part of the group again, and ultimately to be part of a "larger cause."[85] Athletes also noted that receiving social support and encouragement from teammates, coaches, family members, and friends was extremely important in facilitating return to sport. During ACL rehabilitation, medical professionals should strive to give frequent positive feedback to athletes, allow them the freedom to progress at their own pace, connect them with other athletes who have previously suffered ACL injuries, and ensure that they are staying engaged with their teammates, training partners, and coaches.

Considerations for Women

The fundamental core of human motivation and basic psychological needs per SDT is widely considered to be invariant across gender.[100] However, some smaller differences in sources of motivation among males and females have been noted. Multiple studies have found gender differences in intrinsic and extrinsic motivation among young adults, athletes, students, and elderly populations.[106–108] In each of these studies, data suggest that women have higher levels of intrinsic motivation and identified regulation than males, as well as lower levels of external regulation. However, the gender differences in intrinsic versus extrinsic motivation in the athlete sample (369 competitive swimmers) were

considered marginal.[106] Another literature suggests that across domains, women tend to be more motivated by the idea of mastering tasks and self-improvement, whereas men tend to be more motivated by external incentives.[109] This suggests that male athletes recovering from ACLR may be more motivated to return to sport by financial incentives or external recognition than women, who may be more motivated to return to sport by the idea of getting back to their old self and regaining a sense of competence in their sport. While further speculation is possible, more research is needed to determine whether significant gender differences exist among athletes in terms of intrinsic versus extrinsic motivation for returning to sport following ACLR. SDT posits that the satisfaction of basic psychological needs is fundamental to intrinsic motivation in both men and women. Thus medical professionals should focus on supporting athletes' needs for autonomy, relatedness, and competence, regardless of gender.

Research suggests that creating an autonomy-supporting environment for individuals recovering from orthopedic injuries is important. In such an environment, medical professionals provide athletes with different options and opportunities to choose from. They show athletes respect and acknowledge their emotions and opinions, and they provide meaningful rationales behind treatment recommendations.[96] While gender differences were not examined, one study suggests that when physical therapists supported their patients' (who have undergone ACLR) needs for autonomy in these ways, it led to higher levels of intrinsic motivation and, subsequently, greater adherence to prescribed at-home exercises.[102] Regarding relatedness, some research suggests that women possess a higher drive to affiliate with others and are often more invested in interpersonal relationships than men.[110] Medical professionals working with female athletes recovering from ACLR should work to harness motivation stemming from a desire to reintegrate into the social atmosphere offered by one's team. Further research should examine the extent to which gender differences exist in the satisfaction of basic psychological needs among athletes recovering from ACLR in an effort to aid practitioners in bolstering their patients' psychological needs throughout rehabilitation.

Measures

The Treatment Self-Regulation Questionnaire (TSRQ)[111] was originally designed to assess autonomous and controlled reasons for adhering to a weight loss program but has since been adapted to assess motivation to adhere to medical treatments among patients with diabetes, participants in a smoking cessation intervention, and, notably, patients recovering from ACLR.[97,102,112] The original questionnaire was used at multiple time points throughout a weight loss program with question stems including "I am staying in the weight loss program because…" and "I have been following the guidelines of the program because…".[111] Example items assessing externally regulated motivation include "I want others to see that I am really trying to lose weight," and "I'll feel like a failure if I don't." Example items assessing more autonomous motivation include "It's important to me personally to succeed in losing weight" and "I believe it's the best way to help myself." Each reason is rated on a five-point Likert scale ranging from "not true at all" to "very true." The TSRQ has shown acceptable validity and reliability across multiple settings and health behaviors and can be easily modified to assess ACLR recovery.[113]

Consistent with SDT, it is important to assess the satisfaction of basic psychological needs along with motivation. A number of studies have measured basic psychological needs in specific contexts, including work and relationships, whereas others have examined the general satisfaction of psychological needs.[114–117] The Basic Needs Satisfaction in General Scale (BNSG-S) consists of 21 items that assess the general satisfaction of basic psychological needs for autonomy (e.g., "I feel like I am free to decide for myself how I live my life," "I generally feel free to express my ideas and opinions"), competence (e.g., "People I know tell me I am good at what I do," "Most days I feel a sense of accomplishment from what I do"), and relatedness (e.g., "People in my life care about me," "I really like the people I interact with"). Items are rated on a seven-point Likert scale from "not at all true" to "very true." The BNSG-S may yield clinically useful information about the extent to which patients' basic psychological needs are satisfied in general. However, some research has questioned the psychometric properties of the BNSG-S, with potential issues including low reliability for the autonomy and competence scales.[118]

As no current measures exist to evaluate basic psychological needs during recovery from sports injuries, medical professionals may consider using the Basic Needs Satisfaction in Sport Scale[119] to assess psychological needs satisfaction in the domain of sport more broadly. Data suggest that greater psychological needs satisfaction in sport is positively associated with mental toughness and positive affect,[120] both of which are helpful during ACLR rehabilitation. In addition, it would be important for medical professionals to understand the extent to which injured athletes' psychological needs were satisfied in their sport, but were

unsatisfied during rehabilitation. It is clear that sports participation confers a number of psychological benefits for those involved, but the loss of the ability to participate in one's sport may result in a loss of basic psychological needs satisfaction and a subsequent decrease in motivation to return to one's sport. Future research should examine alternative means for athletes to satisfy their basic psychological needs throughout rehabilitation, especially for athletes whose psychological needs were satisfied primarily via active sport participation.

HOW CAN SPORT PSYCHOLOGISTS HELP?

This chapter has discussed the role of mood disturbance, anxiety, fear of reinjury, locus of control, self-efficacy, self-confidence, motivation, and self-determination on the return to play process following ACL injury. Identification of these underlying psychological difficulties that can impede the return to play process by the physician is important to facilitate appropriate referrals to sport psychologists and/or other resources who may assist athletes in returning to play sooner following ACL injuries. Specifically, sport psychologists are able to provide a multitude of interventions that are individualized to the athlete and their particular situation as part of the recovery process. These interventions may include, for example, building specific psychological skills, addressing personal issues that could be interfering with the recovery process, collaborating with the patient's family to facilitate appropriate social support, learning better ways to cope with stress, and teaching achievement-oriented skills. Essentially, the sports psychologist can help individuals better understand the relationship between experiences in recovery and other aspects of their life to facilitate personal development and increase the patient's perceptions of control over their recovery.

Sport psychologists typically work one-on-one with patients to address areas of concern. For example, fear of reinjury and/or depression may be focused on, with sessions including education, normalization, introduction, and application of interventions and termination from treatment. Many psychological interventions are available, though, a specific intervention is cognitive behavior therapy (CBT) to help patients recognize and replace patterns of maladaptive thoughts, behaviors, and emotions. As part of CBT, psychologists will employ strategies such as disputing in order to guide patients to review evidence that will falsify the maladaptive thoughts and make alternative thoughts based on available evidence. In some cases, goal setting may also be incorporated to help patients set realistic expectations for their recovery and different milestones (e.g., engaging in physical activity). Throughout this process, the sports psychologist ultimately serves as part of the patient's social support network and aims to give patients the tools to satisfy their three basic psychological needs to foster motivation, adherence to rehabilitation, decreased physical/psychological symptoms, well-being, and health.

REFERENCES

1. Majewski M, Susanne H, Klaus S. Epidemiology of athletic knee injuries: a 10-year study. *Knee.* 2006;13:184–188.
2. Kvist J. Rehabilitation following anterior cruciate ligament injury: current recommendations for sports participation. *Sports Med.* 2004;34(4):269–280.
3. Ardern CL, Webster KE, Taylor NF, Feller JA. Return to sport following anterior cruciate ligament reconstruction surgery: a systematic review and meta-analysis of the state of play. *Br J Sports Med.* 2011;45:596–606.
4. Ardern CL, Taylor NF, Feller JA, Whitehead TS, Webster KE. Sports participation 2 years after anterior cruciate ligament reconstruction in athletes who had not returned to sport at 1 year: a prospective follow-up of physical function and psychological factors in 122 athletes. *Am J Sports Med.* 2015;43(4):848–856.
5. Feller JA, Webster KE. A randomized comparison of patellar tendon and hamstring tendon anterior cruciate ligament reconstruction. *Am J Sports Med.* 2003;31(4):564–573.
6. Ardern CL, Taylor NF, Feller JA, Webster KE. Fifty-five per cent return to competitive sport following anterior cruciate ligament reconstruction surgery: an updated systematic review and meta-analysis including aspects of physical functioning and contextual factors. *Br J Sports Med.* 2014;48:1543–1552.
7. Moezy A, Olyaei G, Hadian M, Razi M, Faghihzadeh S. A comparative study of whole body vibration training and conventional training on knee proprioception and postural stability after anterior cruciate ligament reconstruction. *Br J Sports Med.* 2008;42:373–378.
8. Risberg MA, Mork M, Jenssen HK, Holm I. Design and implementation of a neuromuscular training program following anterior cruciate ligament reconstruction. *J Orthop Sports Phys Ther.* 2001;31(11):620–631.
9. Heijne A, Axelsson K, Werner S, Biguet G. Rehabilitation and recovery after anterior cruciate ligament reconstruction: patients' experiences. *Scan J Med Sci Sports.* 2007;18(3):325–335.
10. Langford JL, Webster KE, Feller JA. A prospective longitudinal study to assess psychological changes following anterior cruciate ligament reconstruction surgery. *Br J Sports Med.* 2008;43:377–381.
11. Ardern CL, Taylor NF, Feller JA, Whitehead TS, Webster KE. Psychological responses matter in returning to preinjury level of sport after anterior cruciate ligament reconstruction surgery. *Am J Sports Med.* 2013;41(7):1549–1558.
12. Kvist J, Ek A, Sporrstedt K, Good L. Fear of re-injury: a hindrance for returning to sports after anterior cruciate ligament reconstruction. *Knee Surg Sports Traumatol Arthrosc.* 2005;13:393–397.
13. Webster KE, Feller JA, Lambros C. Development and preliminary validation of a scale to measure the psychological impact of returning to sport following anterior cruciate ligament reconstruction surgery. *Phys Ther Sport.* 2008;9:9–15.
14. Brewer BW. The role of psychological factors in sport injury rehabilitation outcomes. *Int Rev Sport Exerc Psychol.* 2010;3(1):40–61.
15. Christino MA, Fantry AJ, Vopat BG. Psychological aspects of recovery following anterior cruciate ligament reconstruction. *J Am Acad Orthop Surg.* 2015;23:501–509.
16. Forsdyke D, Smith A, Jones M, Gledhill A. Psychosocial factors associated with outcomes of sports injury rehabilitation in competitive athletes: a mixed studies systematic review. *Behav Theor.* 2015;50:537–544.
17. Ardern CL. Anterior cruciate ligament reconstruction—not exactly a one-way ticket back to the preinjury level: a review of contextual factors affecting return to sport after surgery. *Am J Sports Med.* 2015;7(3):224–230.
18. Roos HP, Ornell M, Gardsell P, Lohmander L, Lindstrand A. Soccer after anterior cruciate ligament injury–an incompatible combination? A national survey of incidence and risk factors and a 7-year follow-up of 310 players. *Acta Orthop Scand.* 1995;66(2):107–112.
19. Shimokochi Y, Shultz SJ. Mechanisms of noncontact anterior cruciate ligament injury. *J Athletic Training.* 2008;43(4):396–408.
20. Morrey MA, Stuart MJ, Smith AM, Wiese-Bjornstal DM. A longitudinal examination of athletes' emotional and cognitive responses to anterior cruciate ligament injury. *Clin J Sport Med.* 1999;9:63–69.
21. Brewer BW, Cornelius AE, Sklar JH, et al. Pain and negative mood during rehabilitation after anterior cruciate ligament reconstruction: a daily process analysis. *Scan J Med Sci Sports.* 2007;17:520–529.
22. Watson D, Clark LA. Negative affectivity: the disposition to experience aversive emotional states. *Psychol Bull.* 1984;96(3):465.
23. Brewer BW. Self-identity and specific vulnerability to depressed mood. *J Personal.* 1993;61(3):343–364.
24. Cyranowski JM, Frank E, Young E, Shear K. Adolescent onset of the gender difference in lifetime rates of major depression: a theoretical model. *Arch Gen Psychiatry.* 2000;51:21–27.
25. Nolen-Hoeksema S. Gender differences in depression. *Curr Dir Psychol Sci.* 2001;10(5):173–176.

26. Kendler KS, Prescott CA. A population-based twin study of lifetime major depression in men and women. *Arch Gen Psychiat*. 1999;56.

27. Smith AN, Stuart MJ, Wiese-Bjornstal DM, Miliner EK, O'Fallon WM, Crowson CS. Competitive athletes: pre-injury and postinjury mood state and self-esteem. *Mayo Clinic Proceedings*. Vol. 68. Elsevier; 1993.

28. Appaneal RN, Levine BR, Perna FM, Roh JL. Measuring postinjury depression among male and female competitive athletes. *J Sport Exerc Psychol*. 2009;31:60–76.

29. Storch EA, Storch JB, Killiany EM, Roberti JW. Self-reported psychopathology in athletes: a comparison of intercollegiate student-athletes and non-athletes. *J Sport Behav*. 2005;28(1):86–98.

30. Yang J, Peek-Asa C, Corlette JD, Cheng G, Foster DT, Albright J. Prevalence of and risk factors associated with symptoms of depression in competitive collegiate student athletes. *Clin J Sport Med*. 2007;17(6):481–487.

31. Smith AM, Scott SG, O'Fallon WM, Young ML. Emotional responses of athletes to injury. *Mayo Clin Proc*. 1990;65(1):38–50.

32. Pollock V, Cho DW, Reker D, Volavka J. Profile of Mood States: the factors and their psychological correlates. *J Nerv Ment Disord*. 1979;167(10):612–614.

33. Dawes H, Roach NK. Emotional responses of athletes to injury and treatment. *Physiotherapy*. 1997;83(5):243–247.

34. Berger BG, Motl RW. Exercise and mood: a selective review and synthesis of research employing the profile of mood states. *J Appl Sport Psychol*. 2008;12(1):69–92.

35. Curran S, Andrykowski MA, Studts JL. Short form of the profile of mood states (POMS-SF): psychometric information. *Psychol Assess*. 1995;7(1):80–83.

36. Cella DF, Jacobsen PB, Orav EJ, Holland JC, Silberfarb PM, Rafla S. A brief POMS measure of distress for cancer patients. *J Chronic Dis*. 1987;40(10):939–942.

37. Shacham S. A shortened version of the profile of mood states. *J Pers Assess*. 1983;47(3):305–306.

38. Mainwaring LM, Hutchison M, Bisschop SM, Comper P, Richards DW. Emotional response to sport concussion compared to ACL injury. *Brian Inj*. 2010;24(4):589–597.

39. Tripp DA, Stanish W, Ebel-Lam A, Brewer BW, Birchard J. Fear of reinjury, negative affect, and catastrophizing predicting return to sport in recreational athletes with anterior cruciate ligament injuries at 1 year postsurgery. *Rehabil Psychol*. 2007;52(1):74–81.

40. Flanigan DC, Everhart JS, Pedroza AD, Smith TO, Kaeding CC. Fear of reinjury (kinesiophobia) and persistent knee symptoms are common factors for lack of return to sport after anterior cruciate ligament reconstruction. *Arthroscopy*. 2013;29(8):1322–1329.

41. Miller RP, Kori S, Todd D. The Tampa scale: a measure of kinesiophobia. *Clin J Pain*. 1991;7(10):51–52.

42. Vlaeyen JW, Kole-Snijders AM, Boeren RG, van Eek H. Fear of movement/(re)injury in chronic low back pain and its relation to behavioral performance. *Pain*. 1995;62(3):363–372.

43. Johnston LH, Carroll D. The context of emotional responses to athletic injury: a qualitative analysis. *J Sport Rehabil*. 1998;7:206–220.

44. Ardern CL, Taylor NF, Feller JA, Webster KE. Return-to-sport outcomes at 2 to 7 years after anterior cruciate ligament reconstruction surgery. *Am J Sports Med*. 2012;40(1):41–48.

45. Leeuw M, Goossens MEJB, Linton SJ, Crombez G, Boersma K, Vlaeyen JW. The fear-avoidance model of musculoskeletal pain: current state of scientific evidence. *J Behav Med*. 2006;30(1):77–94.

46. McLean CP, Anderson ER. Brave men and timid women? A review of the gender differences in fear and anxiety. *Clin Psychol Rev*. 2009;29:496–505.

47. Anderson JC, Williams S, McGee R, Silva PA. DSM-III disorders in preadolescent children: prevalence in a large sample from the general population. *Arch Gen Psychiatry*. 1987;44(69–76).

48. Ollendick TH. Reliability and validity of the revised fear survey schedule for children (FSSC-R). *Behav Res Ther*. 1983;21(6):685–692.

49. Muris P, Ollendick TH. The assessment of contemporary fears in adolescents using a modified version of the fear survey schedule for children-revised. *J Anxiety Disord*. 2002;16:567–584.

50. Bruce SE, Yonkers KA, Otto MW, et al. Influence of psychiatric comorbidity on recovery and recurrence in generalized anxiety disorder, social phobia, and panic disorder: a 12-year prospective study. *Am J Psychiat*. 2005;162:1179–1187.

51. Menzies RG, Clarke JC. The etiology of phobias: a non-associative account. *Clin Psychol Rev*. 1995;15(1):23–48.

52. Thorpe SJ, Salkovskis PM. Phobic beliefs: do cognitive factors play a role in specific phobias? *Behav Res Ther*. 1995;33(7):805–816.

53. Wood W, Eagly AH. A cross-cultural analysis of the behavior of women and men: implications for the origins of sex differences. *Psychol Bull*. 2002;128(5):699–727.

54. Ross CE, Mirowsky J. Age and the gender gap in the sense of personal control. *Soc Psychol Q*. 2002;65(2):125–145.

55. Buchanan TNS. Race and gender differences in self-efficacy: assessing the role of gender role attitudes and family background. *Sex Roles*. 2008;58:822–836.

56. Blagden JC, Craske MG. Effects of active and passive rumination and distraction: a pilot replication with anxious mood. *J Anxiety Disord*. 1996;10(4):243–252.

57. Podlog L, Eklund RC. Return to sport after serious injury: a retrospective examination of motivation and psychological outcomes. *J Sport Rehabil*. 2005;14:20–34.

58. Crombez G, Vlaeyen JW, Heuts PH, Lysens R. Pain-related fear is more disabling than pain itself: evidence on the role of pain-related fear in chronic back pain disability. *Pain*. 1999;80(1–2):329–339.

59. Nederhand MJ, Ijzerman MJ, Hermans HJ, Turk DC, Zilvold G. Predictive value of fear avoidance in developing chronic neck pain disability: consequences for clinical decision making. *Arch Phys Med Rehabil*. 2004;85(3):496–501.

60. Woby SR, Roach NK, Urmston M, Watson PJ. Psychometric properties of the TKS-11: a shortened version of the Tampa scale for kinesiophobia. *Pain*. 2005;117(1–2):137–144.
61. Wallston KA, Wallston BS, DeVellis R. Development of the multidimensional health locus of control (MHLC) scales. *Health Educ Monogr*. 1978;6(2):160–170.
62. Seeman M, Evans JW. Alienation and learning in a hospital setting. *Am Sociol Rev*. 1962;27(6):772–782.
63. Coan RW. Personality variables associated with cigarette smoking. *J Pers Social Psychol*. 1973;26(1):86–104.
64. Balch P, Ross AW. Predicting success in weight reduction as a function of locus of control: a unidimensional and multidimensional approach. *J Consult Clin Psychol*. 1975;43(1):119.
65. Wallston KA, Kaplan GD, Maides SA. Development and validation of the health locus of control (HLC) scale. *J Consult Clin Psychol*. 1976;44(4):580–585.
66. Burish TG, Carey MP, Wallston KA, Stein MJ, Jamison RN, Lyles JN. Health locus of control and chronic disease: an external orientation may be advantageous. *J Soc Clin Psychol*. 1984;2(4):326–332.
67. Kluge CA, McAleer CA. Factors that predict successful outcome in a cancer-rehabilitation program–a pilot study. *Rehabil Couns Bull*. 1978;21(3):246–252.
68. Norman P. Health locus of control and health behaviour: an investigation into the role of health value and behaviour-specific efficacy beliefs. *Personal Individ Differ*. 1995;18(2):213–218.
69. Cousins SOB. Exercise cognition among elderly women. *J Appl Sport Psychol*. 1994;8(2):131–145.
70. Wallston KA. Hocus-pocus, the focus isn't strictly on locus: Rotter's social learning theory modified for health. *Cog Ther Res*. 1992;16(2):183–199.
71. Bandura A. Self-efficacy: toward a unifying theory of behavioral change. *Psychol Rev*. 1977;84(2):191–215.
72. Scholz U, Sniehotta FF, Schwarzer R. Predicting physical exercise in cardiac rehabilitation: the role of phase-specific self-efficacy beliefs. *J Sport Exerc Psychol*. 2005;27(2):135–151.
73. Altmaier EM, Russell DW, Kao CF, Lehmann TR, Weinstein JN. Role of self-efficacy in rehabilitation outcome among chronic low back pain patients. *J Couns Psychol*. 1993;40(3):335–339.
74. Robinson-Smith G, Johnston MV, Allen J. Self-care self-efficacy, quality of life, and depression after stroke. *Arch Phys Med Rehabil*. 2000;81(4):460–464.
75. Milne M, Hall C, Forwell L. Self-efficacy, imagery use, and adherence to rehabilitation by injured athletes. *J Sport Rehabil*. 2005;14:150–167.
76. Chmielewski TL, Jones D, Day T, Tillman SM, Lentz TA, George SZ. The association of pain and fear of movement/reinjury with function during anterior cruciate ligament reconstruction rehabilitation. *J Orthop Sports Phys Ther*. 2008;38(12):746–753.
77. Thomeé P, Währborg P, Börjesson M, Thomeé R, Eriksson BI, Karlsson J. Self-efficacy of knee function as a pre-operative predictor of outcome 1 year after anterior cruciate ligament reconstruction. *Knee Surg Sports Traumatol Arthrosc*. 2008;16:118–127.
78. Thomeé P, Währborg P, Börjesson M, Thomeé R, Eriksson BI, Karlsson J. Determinants of self-efficacy in the rehabilitation of patients with anterior cruciate ligament injury. *J Rehabil Med*. 2007;39:486–492.
79. Feltz DL. Self-confidence and sports performance. *Exerc Sport Sci Rev*. 1988;16:423–457.
80. Woodman T, Hardy L. The relative impact of cognitive anxiety and self-confidence upon sport performance: a meta-analysis. *J Sport Sci*. 2003;21(6):443–457.
81. Besharat MA, Pourbohlool S. Moderating effects of self-confidence and sport self-efficacy on the relationship between competitive anxiety and sport performance. *Psychol*. 2011;2(7):760–765.
82. Koivula N, Hassmen P, Fallby J. Self-esteem and perfectionism in elite athletes: effects on competitive anxiety and self-confidence. *Personal Individ Differ*. 2002;32:865–875.
83. LaMott EE. *The Anterior Cruciate Ligament Injured Athlete: The Psychological Process* (unpublished PhD thesis). University of Minnesota; 1994.
84. Taylor J, Taylor S. *Psychological Approaches to Sport Injury Rehabilitation*. Gaithersburg, MD: Aspen Publication; 1997:273.
85. Podlog L, Eklund RC. A longitudinal investigation of competitive athletes' return to sport following serious injury. *J Appl Sport Psych*. 2006;18(1):44–68.
86. Carson F, Polman RCJ. ACL injury rehabilitation: a psychological case study of a professional rugby union player. *J Clin Sport Psych*. 2008;2:71–90.
87. Maccoby EE, Jacklin CN. *The Psychology of Sex Differences*. Vol. 2. Stanford University Press; 1978.
88. Lirgg CD. Gender differences in self-confidence in physical activity: a meta-analysis of recent studies. *J Sport Exerc Psychol*. 1991;8:294–310.
89. Sanguinetti C, Lee AM, Nelson J. Reliability estimates and age and gender comparisons of expectations of success in sex-typed activities. *J Sport Psychol*. 1985;7:379–388.
90. Solmon MA, Lee AM, Belcher D, Harrison Jr L, Wells L. Beliefs about gender appropriateness, ability, and competence in physical activity. *J Teach Phys Educ*. 2003;22:261–279.
91. Corbin CB, Landers DM, Feltz DL, Senior K. Sex differences in performance estimates: female lack of confidence vs. male boastfulness. *Res Q Exerc Sport*. 1983;54(4):407–410.
92. Waldrop D. *Perceived Competence, Self-efficacy, and Optimism in Recovery from Orthopedic Surgery: The Role of General and Specific Expectancies* (dissertation). Ann Arbor, MI: University of Memphis; 1999.
93. Thomeé P, Währborg P, Börjesson M, Thomeé R, Eriksson BI, Karlsson J. A new instrument for measuring self-efficacy in patients with an anterior cruciate ligament injury. *Scan J Med Sci Sports*. 2006;16:181–187.

94. Waldrop D, Lightsey OR, Ethington CA, Woemmel CA, Coke AL. Self-efficacy, optimism, health competence, and recovery from orthopedic surgery. *J Couns Psychol.* 2001;48(2):233–238.

95. Mohtadi N. Development and validation of the Quality of Life Outcome Measure (Questionnaire) for chronic anterior cruciate ligament deficiency. *Am J Sports Med.* 1998;26(3):350–359.

96. Williams GC, Freedman ZR, Deci EL. Supporting autonomy to motivate patients with diabetes for glucose control. *Diabetes Care.* 1998;21(10):1644–1651.

97. Williams GC, Gagné M, Ryan RM, Deci EL. Facilitating autonomous motivation for smoking cessation. *Health Psychol.* 2002;21(1):40–50.

98. Duda JL, Smart AE, Tappe MK. Predictors of adherence in the rehabilitation of athletic injuries: an application of personal investment theory. *J Sport Exerc Psych.* 1989;11:367–381.

99. Brewer BW, Cornelius AE, Van Raalte JL, et al. Protection motivation theory and adherence to sport injury rehabilitation revisited. *Sport Psychol.* 2003;17:95–103.

100. Deci EL, Ryan RM. The "what" and "why" of goal pursuits: human needs and the self-determination of behavior. *Psychol Inq.* 2000;11(4):227–268.

101. Deci EL, Ryan RM. The general causality orientations scale: self-determination in personality. *J Res Personal.* 1985;19:109–134.

102. Chan DK, Lonsdale C, Yung PS, Chan KM. Patient motivation and adherence to postsurgery rehabilitation exercise recommendations: the influence of physiotherapists' autonomy-supportive behaviors. *Arch Phys Med Rehabil.* 2009;90:1977–1982.

103. Ryan RM, Deci EL. The darker and brighter sides of human existence: basic psychological needs as a unifying concept. *Psychol Inq.* 2000;11(4):319–338.

104. Bianco T, Malo S, Orlick T. Sport injury and illness: elite skiers describe their experiences. *Res Q Exerc Sport.* 1999;70(2):157–169.

105. Podlog L, Eklund RC. Assisting injured athletes with the return to sport transition. *Clin J Sport Med.* 2004;14(5):257–259.

106. Pelletier LG, Fortier MS, Vallerand RJ, Tuson KM, Brière NM, Blais MR. Toward a new measure of intrinsic motivation, extrinsic motivation, and amotivation in sports: the Sport Motivation Scale (SMS). *J Sport Exerc Psychol.* 1995;17:35–53.

107. Vallerand RJ, Pelletier LG, Blais MR, Brière NM, Senécal C, Vallières EF. The academic motivation scale: a measure of intrinsic, extrinsic, and amotivation in education. *Educ Psychol Meas.* 1992;52:1003–1016.

108. Vallerand RJ, O'Connor BP. Motivation in the elderly: a theoretical framework and some promising findings. *Can Psychol.* 1989;30(3):538–550.

109. Duda JL. The relationship between goal perspectives, persistence, and behavioral intensity among male and female recreational sport participants. *Leis Sci.* 1988;10(2):95–106.

110. Kirsh GA, Kuiper NA. Individualism and relatedness themes in the context of depression, gender, and a self-schema model of emotion. *Can Psychol.* 2002;43(2):76–90.

111. Williams GC, Grow VM, Freedman ZR, Ryan RM, Deci EL. Motivational predictors of weight loss and weight-less maintenance. *J Pers Social Psychol.* 1996;70(1).

112. Williams GC, McGregor HA, Zeldman A, Freedman ZR, Deci EL. Testing a self-determination theory process model for promoting glycemic control through diabetes self-management. *Health Psychol.* 2004;23(1):58–66.

113. Levesque CS, Williams GC, Elliot D, Pickering MA, Bodenhamer B, Finley PJ. Validating the theoretical structure of the Treatment Self-Regulation Questionnaire (TSRQ) across three different health behaviors. *Health Educ Res.* 2007;22(5):691–702.

114. Deci EL, Ryan RM, Gagné M, Leone DR, Usunov J, Kornazheva BP. Need satisfaction, motivation, and well-being in the work organizations of a former Eastern bloc country: a cross-cultural study of self-determination. *Pers Soc Psychol Bull.* 2001;27(8):930–942.

115. La Guardia JG, Ryan RM, Couchman CE, Deci EL. Within-person variation in security of attachment: a self-determination theory perspective on attachment, need fulfillment, and well-being. *J Pers Social Psychol.* 2000;79(3).

116. Gagné M. The role of autonomy support and autonomy orientation in prosocial behavior engagement. *Motiv Emot.* 2003;27(3):199–223.

117. Kashdan TB, Julian T, Merritt K, Uswatte G. Social anxiety and posttraumatic stress in combat veterans: relations to well-being and character strengths. *Behav Res Ther.* 2006;44:561–583.

118. Johnston MM, Finney SJ. Measuring basic needs satisfaction: evaluating previous research and conducting new psychometric evaluations of the basic needs satisfaction in general scale. *Contemp Educ Psychol.* 2010;35:280–296.

119. Ng JYY, Lonsdale C, Hodge K. The basic needs satisfaction in sport scale (BNSSS): instrument development and initial validity evidence. *Psychol Sport Exerc.* 2011;12:257–264.

120. Mahoney JW, Gucciardi DF, Ntoumanis N, Mallett CJ. Mental toughness in sport: motivational antecedents and associations with performance and psychological health. *J Sport Exerc Psychol.* 2014;36(3):281–292.

Index

Note: Page numbers followed by "f" indicate figures, "t" indicate tables.

Printed in the United States
By Bookmasters